Alternative Medicine

Alternative Medicine

A Bibliography of Books in English

COMPILED BY

Ruth West and Joanna E. Trevelyan

Mansell Publishing Limited
LONDON   NEW YORK

First published 1985 by Mansell Publishing Limited
(A subsidiary of The H.W. Wilson Company)
6 All Saints Street, London N1 9RL, England
950 University Avenue, Bronx, New York 10452, U.S.A.

British Library Cataloguing in Publication Data

West, Ruth
    Alternative medicine: a bibliography of books in English.
    1. Therapeutic systems—Bibliography
    I. Title   II. Trevelyan, Joanna E.
    016.6155   Z6665.A1

    ISBN 0-7021-1721-6

Library of Congress Cataloging in Publication Data

West, Ruth, 1948–
    Alternative medicine.

    Includes index.
    1. Therapeutics, Physiological--Bibliography.
I. Trevelyan, Joanna E. [DNLM: 1. Holistic Health--bibliography.
2. Therapeutic Cults--bibliography. ZWB 890 W519a]
Z6665. P49W47 1985 [RM700] 016.6155 84-27181
ISBN 0-7201-1721-6

Printed and bound in Great Britain

Contents

Foreword

This book should help dispel the nonsensical ideas that natural medicine relies more on instinct than intellect and that as it has no literature it cannot be a valid subject.

The financial resources available to the different natural medical disciplines are insignificantly small as compared with those for allopathic, orthodox medicine. Many of the therapies rely to a certain degree on the experience and the publications of countries other than the United Kingdom: acupuncture, for example, on China and Japan, homoeopathy on India and Greece, chiropractic on North America. In the United Kingdom itself scarcely any money is available for research, or for practitioners and theoreticians to sit back free from the day-to-day pressures of practice to consider their subjects. Thus it is a measure of authors' enthusiasm and dedication that so much has in fact been written.

This bibliography draws together for the first time, I believe, the works in English relating to six important systems of treatment: Chinese medicine and acupuncture, chiropractic, herbal medicine, homoeopathy, naturopathy and clinical nutrition, and osteopathy. The range covered is wide: in terms of weight from pamphlets to substantial books, in time from the eighteenth century and earlier to the present day, in scholarship from slim, practical, self-help manuals to the most careful researches of sinology. No reference is made to the many thousands of articles published in different journals each year.

The map of the living disciplines of natural medicine can never be fixed in an irrevocably definitive way, nor allow for their growth, revision or change in emphasis, but this volume comes as close as is practical to realizing such an aim.

Roger Hill MA, BAc
Joint Convenor, Council for
Complementary and Alternative
Medicine

Introduction

Gaining access to sources of information about any newly expanding area of knowledge is rarely an easy task. Alternative medicine, we were warned, would prove no exception. Our advisers were right.

Our first difficulty was to establish what is meant by alternative medicine. Different organizations and causes all seem to have their own criteria for inclusion or exclusion of the various unorthodox therapies that can be found. Some, for example, talk of only four or five alternative (or as they prefer to call them, 'complementary') therapies; others—including the World Health Organization—consider that alternatives should cover all forms of health care provision that 'usually lie outside the official health sector', from Ayurvedic medicine (indigenous to India) to tribal medicine 'and even Christian Science'. To have accepted this definition would have meant a bibliography covering some sixty or more different therapies.

The extent to which these various views have confused and/or misled people was brought home to us when we looked at the results of a recent survey of the public's knowledge of and attitudes towards alternative medicine. Only 46 percent of adults had heard of it 'and/or were able to mention spontaneously a particular type'. And by alternative medicine they meant anything from 'natural things' to 'home remedies', 'health foods', 'more preventive than curing', and 'private medicine'. The only actual therapies mentioned were herbal medicine, homoeopathy, acupuncture and osteopathy.

We decided to aim at simplifying rather than complicating matters by including only those therapies that are of international standing and provide full-time training courses. This is not to say that we consider that the remaining sixty or so are not of any value, for such a judgement is not our task. Rather, we hope that they will be covered in subsequent bibliographies.

Our second—and major—difficulty came when we began to locate and list books. We thought first to check with the main library classification systems in the hope that they would be able to help us.

They could not. None of them listed all the major therapies under alternative medicine; for example, we found therapies listed under such disparate headings as 'tribal medicine' and 'biotechnology'. The systems also required prior knowledge of the subject by the user if they were to be of any worthwhile assistance. So for our bibliography we turned instead to specialist sources for information. These were mainly of five types: specialist libraries, private collections, specialist publishers, specialist booksellers and resource centres. It is from these five types of source, in Britain and the United States, that we compiled the major part of the bibliography. In addition, though, we collected catalogues from British and American publishers in order to pick up the odd book produced by firms not normally associated with alternative medicine. As a further check we consulted specialists in each field to ensure that we had included the pertinent titles. And of course we consulted the British Library.

If we have a bias in our selection of books it has been to the needs of the consumer. We have become aware of a public need for guidance and information on the subject—something that was confirmed in a report produced by the Council of Europe in the summer of 1984. This underlined the fact that there is a gap in the health care needs of people, left because of a dissatisfaction with and turning away from orthodox medicine. The Council had found that a 'persistent and widespread' body of people are therefore turning to the alternatives. We hope that this bibliography will encourage many more people to find some benefit from the use of alternative therapies.

All the major textbooks currently being used by students in the different therapies are listed, along with useful manuals and reference works for researchers and interested practitioners; a selection of historical and philosophical works; and books written by the 'founders' and subsequent major writers in the field. The books are arranged alphabetically according to author under the heading of the appropriate therapy. Our emphasis in selecting the books has been on listing those that are still in print. Where a book is no longer easily available, we have done our best to find the last edition or impression. We should however point out that the inclusion of a book does not necessarily signify our personal recommendation. Only books published in the English language have been included and most of these originate from Britain or the United States. Where we have commented on a book it has been to indicate its type: whether it is an introduction to the therapy, a textbook, of historical importance, a practical guide and so on; or to explain the content of the book where this is not obvious from its title; or else to recommend any particularly good book.

Our task of compiling the bibliography has been greatly eased by
the guidance and advice of many individuals, organizations and
associations, to whom we are deeply indebted. First and foremost we
would like to thank Jeremy Cherfas for his generosity over the use of
his computer, without which we cannot imagine the book ever
having reached completion. Our grateful thanks also go to: The
Koestler Foundation, the British Homoeopathic Association, the
Homoeopathic Development Foundation, Francis Trehertz, Ains-
worths Homoeopathic Pharmacy, the Faculty of Homoeopathy, Mr.
P. Thomas, the librarians at the British School of Osteopathy, Peter
Hawkins, Colin Dove, Mervyn Waldman, the British College of
Osteopathy and Naturopathy, the librarians at the Anglo-European
College of Chiropractic, Alan Breen, Lilian Scofield and the staff of
Wholefood, Monica Bryant, Leon Chaitow, Roger Newman Turner,
Robert Chris Booksellers, The Herb Society, Thomas Bartram,
Barbara Griggs, George Lewith, Joseph Goodman, Books of India,
East-Asia Books and Arts Co., Planetree Resource Centre, Aslib,
Collets' Chinese Bookshop and Gallery, the College of Traditional
Chinese Acupuncture, Stephen Davies, David A. Phillips, Robert
Buist, Roger Hill, Mr. A. K. Burton, Mr. K. Green, Kenneth
Barlow, Peter Deadman, the International College of Oriental
Medicine UK Ltd., the Vegetarian Centre and Bookshop, the
Community Health Foundation, Gerard House, the McCarrison
Society, Jeffrey Bland, the Australian Natural Therapies Associa-
tion, the Southern School of Natural Therapies, the Whole Health
Programme, the Green Farm Nutrition Centre, Robin Monro,
Georg Wikman, the International College of Natural Health
Science, the East West Academy of Healing Arts and Denise Feild.
The *Journal of Alternative Medicine* and the *Journal of Australian Natural
Therapies* published articles on the bibliography, many publishing
companies and bookshops sent us stock lists and many other people
helped us with advice or suggestions of books to include; our thanks
to all these.

Our hope is that the resultant bibliography will provide a good,
balanced 'first' that is of use to all who have an interest in alternative
medicine.

Books on general aspects of alternative medicine

HOLISTIC HEALTH

Benson, Herbert. *The mind/body effect.* 1981. New York: Berkley Books.

———. *The relaxation response.* 1977. London: Fontana.

———. *Beyond the relaxation response.* 1984. New York: Times Book Co. Inc.

Cousins, Norman. *Anatomy of an illness.* 1981. London: Bantam Books.

Dossey, Larry. *Space, time and medicine.* 1982. Boulder, Colorado: Shambhala.

Hastings, Arthur C. (Ed.). *Health for the whole person: the complete guide to holistic medicine.* 1980. Boulder, Colorado: Westview Press.

Pelletier, Kenneth. *Mind as healer, mind as slayer—a holistic approach to preventing stress disorders.* 1978. London: George Allen & Unwin.

———. *Holistic health—from stress to optimum health.* 1979. New York: Delta.

LeShan, Lawrence. *Holistic health.* 1984. London: Turnstone Press.

CRITIQUES OF MODERN MEDICINE

Abse, Danny. *Medicine on trial.* 1967. London: Aldus Books.

Capra, Fritjof. *The turning point: science, society and the rising culture.* 1982. London: Wildwood House.

Doyal, Lesley. *Political economy of health.* 1979. London: Pluto Press.

Dubos, René. *Mirage of health.* 1959. New York: Harper & Row.

Illich, Ivan. *Limits to medicine: medical nemesis, the expropriation of health.* 1977. Harmondsworth, Middlesex: Penguin Books.

Inglis, Brian. *Diseases of civilisation.* 1981. Sevenoaks: Hodder & Stoughton.

Kennedy, Ian. *The unmasking of medicine.* 1983. London: Paladin Grenada.

McKeown, Thomas. *The role of medicine—dreams, mirage or nemesis?* 1979. Oxford: Basil Blackwell.

Medawar, Charles. *The wrong kind of medicine*. 1984. Sevenoaks, Kent: Hodder & Stoughton.

Melville, Arabella and Colin Johnson. *Cured to death: the effects of prescription drugs*. 1982. London: Martin Secker and Warburg.

INTRODUCTIONS TO ALTERNATIVE MEDICINE

Bannerman, R.H., J. Burton and Ch'en Wen-Chieh. *Traditional medicine and health-care coverage*. 1983. Geneva: World Health Organization.

Eagle, Robert. *Alternative medicine: a guide to the medical underground*. 1978. London: Futura Publications.

Fulder, Stephen. *The handbook of complementary medicine*. 1984. Sevenoaks: Hodder & Stoughton.

Hill, Ann (Ed.). *A visual encyclopaedia of unconventional medicine*. 1979. New York: Crown Publishers.

Inglis, Brian. *Natural medicine*. 1980. London: Fontana.

────── and Ruth West. *The alternative health guide*. 1983. London: Michael Joseph.

Stanway, Andrew. *A guide to natural therapies*. 1982. Harmondsworth, Middlesex: Penguin.

Homoeopathy

1   Adams, Myron H. *A practical guide to homoeopathic treatment: designed and arranged for the use of families, prescribers of limited experience and students of homoeopathy.* 455pp. 1913. Philadelphia, Pennsylvania: Boericke and Tafel.

2   Aggrawal, Y.R. *Comparative study of chronic miasms.* 48pp. 1980. New Delhi, India: Vijay.
    A clearly written review.

3   Aggrawal, Y.R. *Diseases of hair and nails.* 38pp. 1982. New Delhi, India: Vijay.

4   Aggrawal, Y.R. *The dose and its repetition.* 27pp. 1977. New Delhi, India: Vijay.
    Draws widely on classical authorities.

5   Aggrawal, Y.R. *Drug relationship: antidotal and inimical.* 38pp. 1979. New Delhi, India: Vijay.

6   Aggrawal, Y.R. *Homoeopathy in surgery.* 43pp. 1982. New Delhi, India: Vijay.

7   Aggrawal, Y.R. *Materia medica of glandular medicines.* 38pp. 1982. New Delhi, India: Vijay.
    A unique study.

8   Aggrawal, Y.R. *Measles and small-pox.* 32pp. 1980. New Delhi, India: Vijay.

9   Aggrawal, Y.R. *A practical solution to potency problems.* 42pp. 1980. New Delhi, India: Vijay.
    A review.

10   Aggrawal, Y.R. *Symptoms and totality of systems.* 38pp. 1981. New Delhi, India: Vijay.

11   Aggrawal, Y.R. *A treatise on bowel nosodes.* 45pp. 1981. New Delhi, India: Vijay.
Recommended.

12   Aggrawal, Y.R. *What a homoeopath should know.* 46pp. 1982. New Delhi, India: Vijay.

13   Allen, H.C. *Keynotes and characteristics with comparisons of some of the leading remedies of the materia medica.* 388pp. 1982. New Delhi, India: B. Jain.
An indispensable reference work for practitioners.

14   Allen, H.C. *The materia medica of some important nosodes.* 62pp. 1982. New Delhi, India: Vijay.
A very complete account.

15   Allen, H.C. *The materia medica of the nosodes and provings of the X-ray.* 591pp. 1982. New Delhi, India: B. Jain.
A classic work for all practitioners; first published in 1910.

16   Allen, H.C. *The therapeutics of intermittent fever.* 342pp. n.d. New Delhi, India: B. Jain. First published in 1879.
An extremely complete discussion.

17   Allen, J.H. *The chronic miasms.* Volume 1: *Psora and pseudo-psora.* 424pp. 1981. New Delhi, India: B. Jain. Volume 2: *Sycosis.* 424pp. *c.*1910. Originally published in the U.S.A.
An important theoretical work.

18   Allen, J.H. *Diseases and therapeutics of the skin.* 331pp. 1951. Calcutta, India: Sett Dey.
Considered to be the best book available on the subject.

19   Allen, Timothy Field. *The encyclopedia of pure materia medica: a record of the positive effects of drugs upon the healthy human organism.* 12 vols. 1976. New Delhi, India: B. Jain. First published in Philadelphia in 1874 as a ten-volume work with an index.
An essential reference for the practitioner.

20   Allen, T.F. *Handbook of materia medica and homoeopathic therapeutics.*

1174pp. 1983. New Delhi, India: B. Jain. First published in 1889 in
Philadelphia.
Arranged alphabetically.

21   Allen, T.F. *A primer of materia medica for practitioners of homoeopathy.*
415pp. 1982. New Delhi, India: B. Jain. First published *c.*1880 in
Philadelphia.

22   Allen, T.F. (editor). *The principles and practicability of Boenning-
hausen's therapeutic pocket book.* 503pp. 1984. New Delhi, India: B. Jain.
This is a historical classic, first published in the 1840s in America.
This 5th edition includes an introduction by H. A. Roberts and
Annie C. Wilson.

23   Allen, William A. *Repertory to the symptoms of intermittent fever.* n.d.
65pp. New Delhi, India: B. Jain. First published in 1882.

24   Almfett, Gustavus A. *Basic principles of homoeopathy: and the laws
governing physical man and life in matter. A catechism.* 51pp. 1959. Bombay,
India: Roy and Company.

25   Ameke, Wilhelm (translated by Alfred Drysdale, edited by R.E.
Dudgeon). *History of homoeopathy: its origin; its conflicts.* 460pp. 1885.
London: E. Gould.
An excellent account of the early history of homoeopathy.

26   Anderson, D., D. Beugel and D. Chardin. *Homoeopathic remedies
for physicians, laymen and therapists.* 140pp. 1978. Homedale, Pennsylvania: Himalayan International Institute.

27   Arndt, H.R. *First lessons in the symptomatology of leading homoeopathic
remedies.* 271pp. 1904. Philadelphia, Pennsylvania: Boericke and
Tafel.

28   Ashwell, Lawrence T. *Companion to the British and American
homoeopathic pharmacopoeias: arranged in the form of a dictionary.* 200pp.
1890. London: Keene and Aswell.

29   Athalye, V.V. *Forty four years in homoeopathy (therapeutic experiences
with useful hints and observations).* 341pp. 1962. Poona, India: Anath
Vidyarthi Griha Prakashan.

30   Aubin, Michel and Philippa Picard (translated by Pat Campbell

and Robin Campbell). *Homoeopathy for doctor and patient.* 162pp. 1983. Bath, Avon: Ashgrove Press.

31 Baehr, B. (translated by C.J. Hempel). *Science of therapeutics according to the principles of homoeopathy.* Volume 1: 638pp. Volume 2: 752pp. 1883. Philadelphia, Pennsylvania: Boericke and Tafel.

32 Banerjea, Subrata Kumar. *Synoptic memorizer of materia medica.* 322pp. 1980. New Delhi, India: World Homoeopathic Links.

33 Banerjee, N.K. *Homoeopathy in the treatment of gonorrhoea and syphilis.* n.d. 242pp. Calcutta, India: Salzer.

34 Banerjee, N.K. and N. Sinha. *A treatise on homoeopathic pharmacy (for diploma and degree students).* 168pp. 1980. Calcutta, India: New Allen Publishers.

35 Barker, J. Ellis. *Miracles of healing and how they are done. A new path to health.* 402pp. London: The Homoeopathic Publishing Company. First published 1931.

36 Barker, J.E. *My testament of healing.* 333pp. 1947. London: The Homoeopathic Publishing Company. First published 1939.

37 Barthel, Horst. *Synthetic repertory* (3 volumes). Volume 1: *Psychic symptoms.* 1071pp. *c.*1974. Volume 2: *General symptoms.* 715pp. 1978. Heidelberg, W. Germany: Karl F. Haug. Rubrics are in English, French and German, and there are three indices to each volume (separate pagination).
   An indispensable reference book. For volume 3, *see* Klunker, W.

38 Baruch, Emanuel M. *On the relations of antitoxin treatment to homoeopathy. Including a new explanation of the law of 'similia'.* 71pp. 1899. New York: Boericke and Runyon.

39 Bayes, William. *Applied homoeopathy: or, specific restorative medicine.* 171pp. 1871. London: Henry Turner and Co.

40 Bell, James B. *The homoeopathic therapeutics of diarrhoea.* 316pp. 1980. New Delhi, India: World Homoeopathic Links. First published in 1869 in the United Kingdom.

41 Berjeau, J. Ph. *The homoeopathic treatment of syphilis, gonorrhoea,*

spermatorrhoea, and urinary diseases. 256pp. 1983. New Delhi, India: B. Jain. First published in 1930 in Philadelphia.

42   Berridge, E.W. *Complete repertory to the homoeopathic materia medica.* 349pp. n.d. New Delhi, India: B. Jain. First published in 1873 in London.

43   Bhattacharyya, A.K. *Tridosha and homoeopathy: the three cosmic elements in homoeopathy.* 122pp. 1982. Calcutta, India: Kirma KLM.
A thorough examination of the subject.

44   Bhattacharyya, M. *Epitome of homoeopathic practice.* 343pp. 1979. Calcutta, India: M. Bhattacharyya.
An authoritative reference book.

45   Bhattacharyya, M. *External homoeopathic medicine and first aid.* 148pp. 1969. Calcutta, India: M. Bhattacharyya.
A useful and comprehensive summary.

46   Bidwell, Glen Irving. *How to use the repertory, with a practical analysis of forty homoeopathic remedies.* 128pp. n.d. Saffron Walden, Essex: Health Science Press.

47   Bihari, Sultan Alam M. *Homoeopathic insight into cancer: cause, treatment and cure.* 135pp. 1982. New Delhi, India: World Homoeopathic Links.

48   Bihari, Sultan A.M. *Unfathomed regions of homoeopathy: a treatise on radiaesthesia by hair transmission.* 168pp. 1983. New Delhi, India: Aggrawal.
Based on the author's research and practice.

49   Blackie, Margery. *The challenge of homoeopathy: the patient, not the cure.* 247pp. 1984. London: Unwin. First published in 1976 as *The patient not the cure.*
A popular and well written introduction. Includes discussion of homoeopathy today.

50   Blackie, M. (edited by C.K. Elliott and Frank Johnson). *Classical homoeopathy.* Volume 1: *Constitutional prescribing.* 256pp. Volume 2: *Symptomatological prescribing.* 256pp. To be published in 1985. Beaconsfield, Buckinghamshire: Beaconsfield.

51   Blackwood, A.L. *Contagious constitutional and blood diseases.* 367pp. 1910. Philadelphia, Pennsylvania: Boericke and Tafel.

5

52 Blackwood, A.L. *Diseases of the kidneys and nervous diseases.* 354pp. 1979. New Delhi, India: B. Jain. First published in 1913.

53 Blackwood, A.L. *Diseases of the liver, pancreas and ductless glands.* 166pp. 1907. Calcutta, India: Sett Dey. A concise discussion.

54 Blackwood, A.L. *The food tract: Its ailments and disease of the peritoneum.* 367pp. 1980. New Delhi, India: World Homoeopathic Links. First published in 1909.

55 Boenninghausen, C.M.F. von (edited by T.L. Bradford). *The lesser writings of C.M.F. von Boenninghausen.* 350pp. 1979. New Delhi, India: B. Jain. First published in 1908 in Philadelphia. An important work.

56 Boenninghausen, C.M.F. von (translated by J. Laurie and edited by Dr Roth). *Manual of homoeopathic therapeutics intended also as a guide to the study of the materia medica.* 493pp. 1847. London: H. Baillière.

57 Boenninghausen, C.M.F. von and R.G. Miller. *The relationship of remedies and sides of the body.* 63pp. n.d. New Delhi, India: B. Jain. Organized into shorthand tables. This and the above are two independent books combined by the publishers.

58 Boenninghausen, C.M.F. von (translated by C.M. Boger). *A systematic alphabetic repertory of homoeopathic remedies.* 269pp. 1979. New Delhi, India: B. Jain. First published in 1899. Covers the antipsoric, antisyphilitic and antisycotic remedies.

59 Boericke, F.A. and E.P. Anshutz. *The elements of homoeopathy theory, materia medica, practice and pharmacy compiled and arranged from homoeopathic textbooks.* 218pp. 1907. Philadelphia, Pennsylvania: Boericke and Tafel.

60 Boericke, Garth. *A compend of the principles of homoeopathic for students in medicine.* 178pp. 1980. New Delhi, India: B. Jain. First published in 1929.

61 Boericke, William. *A compend of the principles of homoeopathy as taught by Hahnemann and verified by a century of clinical application.* 160pp. 1896. San Francisco, California: Boericke and Runyon.

62 Boericke, W. *Pocket manual of materia medica*. 1105pp. 1984. New Delhi, India: B. Jain. First published in 1927 in Philadelphia. An essential aid to all practitioners. This 9th edition is revised and enlarged with the addition of a repertory by Oscar E. Boericke.

63 Boger, C.M. *Additions to Kent's 'Repertory'*. 105pp. 1981. New Delhi, India: B. Jain.
Only for the serious student or practitioner.

64 Boger, C.M. (translated, compiled and augmented by). *Boenninghausen's characteristics*. 184pp. 1982. New Delhi, India: B. Jain. First published in 1905.
Generally considered the most authoritative work available.

65 Boger, C.M. *Studies in the philosophy of healing*. 124pp. 1964. Calcutta, India: Roysingh.
Essays from the close of the golden age of America homoeopathy.

66 Boger, C.M. *The study of materia medica and taking the case*. 32pp. 1961. Calcutta, India: Roysingh.

67 Boger, C.M. *A synoptic key of the materia medica*. 448pp. 1982. New Delhi, India: B. Jain.
A detailed guide for practitioners.

68 Boger, C.M. *Times of the remedies and moon phases*. 248pp. n.d. Calcutta, India: Salzer.
A useful work.

69 Bonnerot and Bernoville-Fortier (translated by R. K. Mukerji). *Ulcer of the stomach and duodenum with cancer of the stomach and stomatitis*. 74pp. 1982. New Delhi, India: B. Jain.
From articles written in the 1930s.

70 Borland, Douglas M. *Children's types*. 66pp. n.d. London: British Homoeopathic Association.
The best in-depth discussion of five types of children. Helpful for the active prescriber.

71 Borland, D.M. *Digestive drugs*. 96pp. 1982. London: British Homoeopathic Association.
A very useful work.

72   Borland, D.M. *Homoeopathy for mother and infant.* 20pp. n.d.
London: British Homoeopathic Association.
An excellent discussion.

73   Borland, D.M. *Homoeopathy in practice* (edited by K. Priestman).
173pp. 1982. Beaconsfield, Buckinghamshire: Beaconsfield.
An excellent and practical discussion. Borland's essence of
remedies is unequalled.

74   Borland, D.M. *Influenzas.* 20pp. n.d. London: British
Homoeopathic Association.
Good.

75   Borland, D.M. *Pneumonias.* 76pp. 1981. New Delhi, India: B.
Jain. First published *c*.1935 in London.
Exceedingly helpful to practitioners.

76   Borland, D.M. *Some emergencies of general practice.* 38pp. 1979.
Bombay, India: Homoeopathic Medical Publishers.
Covers a wide range of emergencies.

77   Boyd, Hamish. *Introduction to homoeopathic medicine.* 239pp. 1981.
Beaconsfield, Buckinghamshire: Beaconsfield.
A systematic introduction intended for the allopathic physician.

78   Boyd, Linn J. *A study of the simile in medicine.* 421pp. 1936.
Philadelphia, Pennsylvania: Boericke and Tafel.
A painstaking review of the literature.

79   Boyd, W.E. *Research on the low potencies of homoeopathy (an account of
some physical properties indicating activity).* 38pp. 1936. London: William
Heinemann Medical Books.

80   Bradford, Thomas Lindsley. *Index of homoeopathic provings.* 305pp.
1901. Philadelphia, Pennsylvania: Boericke and Tafel.

81   Bradford, T.L. *The life and letters of Dr Samuel Hahnemann.* 529pp.
1895. Philadelphia, Pennsylvania: Boericke and Tafel.
An interesting collection of articles of historical and biographical
interest.

82   Bradford, T.L. *The logic of figures or comparative results of
homoeopathic and other treatments.* 212pp. 1900. Philadelphia, Pennsylvania: Boericke and Tafel.

83   British Homoeopathic Association. *A guide to homoeopathy: rational medicine*. 25pp. 1975. London: British Homoeopathic Association. Introductory.

84   British Homoeopathic Association. *The pharmacist and homoeopathic medicine*. 36pp. 1981. London: British Homoeopathic Association. An aid to pharmacists stocking homoeopathic remedies.

85   British Homoeopathic Association. *The progress of homoeopathy: a series of papers illustrative of the position and prospects of medical science*. 269pp. 1867. London: British Homoeopathic Association.

86   British Homoeopathic Society. *British Pharmacopoeia*. 1882. London: E. Gould. 3rd edition.

87   Breyfogle, Wm.L. *Epitome of homoeopathic medicines*. 377pp. 1869. Philadelphia, Pennsylvania: F.E. Boericke.

88   Broakes, W. (translated and annotated by). *Homoeopathic documents: being the authentic bases of homoeopathy, in its reformed and no longer mystical state, namely the declaration of the German Central Homoeopathic Congress and the propositions of Rau*. 152pp. 1839. London: Thomas Hurst.

89   Brown, D. Dyce. *The permeation of present day medicine by homoeopathy*. 111pp. 1904. London: E. Gould.

90   Bryant, J. *A pocket manual or repertory of homoeopathic medicine*. 352pp. 1851. Philadelphia, Pennsylvania: Boericke and Tafel.

91   Buck, Henry. *Outlines of materia medica, regional symptomatology and clinical dictionary*. 783pp. 1865. London: Leath and Ross.

92   Burnett, J. Compton. *The change of life in women and the ills and ailings incident thereto*. 191pp. n.d. New Delhi, India: Hahnemann Enterprises. First published in 1898 in London.

93   Burnett, J.C. *Curability of cataract with medicines*. 116pp. 1983. New Delhi, India: World Homoeopathic Links. Augmented with the therapeutics of ophthalmic diseases and revised by N.K. Banerjee. First published in 1880 in London.

94   Burnett, J.C. *Curability of tumours by medicines*. 345pp. n.d. New Delhi, India: World Homoeopathic Links. First published in 1893 in London.

9

95 Burnett, J.C. *Delicate, backward, puny, and stunted children: their developmental defects, and physical, mental and moral peculiarities considered as ailments amenable to treatment by medicines.* 168pp. 1983. New Delhi, India: B. Jain. First published in 1890 in London.
A detailed discussion of the remedies which can ameliorate abnormalities in children.

96 Burnett, J.C. *Diseases of the skin: their constitutional nature and cure.* 280pp. 1983. New Delhi, India: B. Jain. First published in 1886 in London.

97 Burnett, J.C. *Diseases of the spleen and their remedies clinically illustrated.* 83pp. 1981. New Delhi, India: B. Jain. First published in 1887 in London.

98 Burnett, J.C. *Diseases of the veins.* 171pp. 1889. London: The Homoeopathic Publishing Co. 3rd edition.

99 Burnett, J.C. *Ecce medicus, or Hahnemann as a man and as a physician and the lessons of his life.* 172pp. 1881. London: The Homoeopathic Publishing Co.

100 Burnett, J.C. *Eight years' experience in the new cure for consumption.* 323pp. 1894. London: The Homoeopathic Publishing Co.

101 Burnett, J.C. *Enlarged tonsils cured by medicines.* 100pp. 1981. New Delhi, India: B. Jain. First published in 1900 in London.

102 Burnett, J.C. *Fevers and blood-poisoning and their treatment, with special reference to the use of pyrogenium.* 56pp. 1981. New Delhi, India: World Homoeopathic Links. First published in 1901 in London.

103 Burnett, J.C. *Fifty reasons for being a homoeopath.* 175pp. 1880. London: The Homoeopathic Publishing Co.
A collection of letters. Recommended.

104 Burnett, J.C. *Greater diseases of the liver: jaundice, gall-stones, enlargements, tumours and cancer: and their treatment.* 244pp. 1982. New Delhi, India: B. Jain. First published in 1895 in London.

105 Burnett, J.C. *Gold as a remedy in disease, notably in some forms of organic heart disease, angina pectoris, melancholy, tedium vitae, scrofula, syphilis, skin disease and as an antidote to the ill effects of mercury.* 162pp. n.d. New Delhi, India: B. Jain. First published in 1879 in London.

106   Burnett, J.C. *Gout and its cure.* 178pp. 1983. New Delhi, India: World Homoeopathic Links. First published in 1895 in London.

107   Burnett, J.C. *The medicinal treatment of diseases of the veins.* 172pp. 1881. London: The Homoeopathic Publishing Co.

108   Burnett, J.C. *Natrum muriaticum as test of drug dynamization.* 84pp. 1878. London: E. Gould.
Excellent.

109   Burnett, J.C. *On fistula and its radical cure by medicines.* 108pp. 1981. New Delhi, India: World Homoeopathic Links. First published in 1894 in London.

110   Burnett, J.C. *On neuralgia: its causes and its remedies, with a chapter on angina pectoris.* 72pp. 1894. London: The Homoeopathic Publishing Co.

111   Burnett, J.C. *On the prevention of hare lip, cleft palate and other congenital defects.* 18pp. 1880. London: The Homoeopathic Publishing Co.

112   Burnett, J.C. *The new cure for consumption by its own virus.* n.d. 339pp. New Delhi, India: World Homoeopathic Links. First published in 1890.
This was the first publication on Bacillinum.

113   Burnett, J.C. *Organ diseases of women, notably enlargements and displacements of the uterus and sterility, considered as curable by medicines.* 156pp. 1896. London: The Homoeopathic Publishing Co.

114   Burnett, J.C. *Ringworm: its constitutional nature and cure.* 126pp. 1981. New Delhi, India: World Homoeopathic Links. First published in 1892 in London.

115   Burnett, J.C. *Supersalinity of the blood.* 1882. London: The Homoeopathic Publishing Co.

116   Burnett, J.C. *Tumours of the breast.* 1888. London: James Epps.

117   Burnett, J.C. *Vaccinosis and its cure by thuja; with remarks on homoeoprophylaxis.* 124pp. 1982. New Delhi, India: World Homoeopathic Links. First published in 1884 in London.

118   Burnett, J.C. *Valvular disease of the heart from a new standpoint.* 1885. London: Leam and Ross.

119   Burt, William H. *Characteristic materia medica.* 541pp. 1980. New Delhi, India: B. Jain.

120   Burt, W.H. *Physiological materia medica.* 992pp. 1980. New Delhi, India: B. Jain. First published in 1881 in America.
A definitive work.

120A   Campbell, Anthony. *The two faces of homoeopathy.* 158pp. 1984. London: Jill Norman.

121   Carleton, Edmund. *Homoeopathy in medicine and surgery.* 311pp. 1982. New Delhi, India: B. Jain.
A well written and unique account first published in 1913.

122   Charette, Gilbert (translated by William J. Webb). *What is homoeopathy? An introduction for physicians and laymen.* 133pp. 1934. London: The Homoeopathic Publishing Co. Also translated into five other languages.

123   Chavanon, Paul and Rene Levannier (translated by Geoffrey A. Dudley). *Emergency homoeopathic first aid.* 160pp. 1982. Wellingborough, Northamptonshire: Thorsons.
A very complete account.

124   Chepmell, Edward C. *A domestic homoeopathy restricted to its legitimate sphere of practice together with rules for diet and regimen.* 410pp. 1859. London: Thomas Sanderson.

125   Choudhury, N.M. *A study of materia medica and repertory.* 1085pp. 1983. New Delhi, India: B. Jain.
One of the best Indian materia medica.

126   Clark, A. Gladstone. *Decachords: a concise guide to the homoeopathic materia medica for students of the Missionary School of Medicine and others.* 118pp. 1968. London: The Missionary School of Medicine. First published in 1925.

127   Clarke, J.H. *Catarrh, colds and grippe, including prevention and cure.* 146pp. n.d. New Delhi, India: B. Jain. First published in 1899 in London.
A useful discussion and historically interesting.

128   Clarke, J.H. *Cholera, diarrhoea and dysentery: homoeopathic prevention and cure.* 88pp. n.d. New Delhi, India: B. Jain.
A useful treatise first published in 1893.

129   Clarke, J.H. *A clinical repertory to the dictionary of materia medica together with repertories of causation, temperaments, clinical relationships and natural relationships.* 346pp. 1979. Saffron Walden, Essex: Health Science Press.

130   Clarke, J.H. *Cold-catching, cold preventing, cold-curing: with a section on influenzas.* 116pp. 1896. London: James Epps.

131   Clarke, J.H. *Constitutional medicine: with especial reference to the three constitutions of Dr. von Grauvogl.* 182pp. 1982. New Delhi, India: B. Jain. First published in 1925 in London.
A rare discussion of this subject.

132   Clarke, J.H. *The cure of tumours by medicine with special reference to cancer nosodes.* 195pp. 1908. London: James Epps.

133   Clarke, J.H. *Dictionary of domestic medicine with a special section on diseases of infants.* 255pp. 1949. London: The Homoeopathic Publishing Co. First published in 1890.
A lay person's guide. This 4th edition was revised by Dr. Dorothy Shepherd.

134   Clarke, J.H. *A dictionary of practical materia medica.* 3 volumes: 3321pp. 1982. Saffron Walden, Essex: Health Science Press. First published in 1900, and revised by the author up until 1935. There have only been reprints since.
The most comprehensive but precise materia medica available. Excellent.

135   Clarke, J.H. *Diseases of the glands and bones.* 170pp. 1894. London: The Homoeopathic Publishing Co.

136   Clarke, J.H. *Diseases of the heart and arteries: their causes, nature and treatment.* 195pp. 1981. New Delhi, India: B. Jain. First published in 1895 in London.

137   Clarke, J.H. *Doctor Skinner's grand characteristics of the materia medica.* 32pp. 1982. New Delhi, India: B. Jain. First published in 1931 in London.

138   Clarke, J.H. *The enthusiasm of homoeopathy: with the story of a great enthusiast.* 51pp. 1907. London: The Homoeopathic Publishing Co.

139   Clarke, J.H. *Gunpowder as a war remedy.* 1971. New Delhi, India: B. Jain. First published in 1915 in London.
A provocative description of a wound remedy.

140   Clarke, J.H. *Haemorrhoids and habitual constipation: their constitutional cure.* 112pp. 1897. London: James Epps.

141   Clarke, J.H. *Homoeopathy explained.* 229pp. n.d. New Delhi, India: B. Jain.
An introductory book first published in 1905 in London.

142   Clarke, J.H. *Indigestion: its causes and cure.* 160pp. n.d. New Delhi, India: B. Jain. First published in 1928 in London.
The nutritional comments are dated but the homoeopathy and cases are interesting.

143   Clarke, J.H. *Life and work of James Compton Burnett.* 142pp. 1904. London: The Homoeopathic Publishing Co.

144   Clarke, J.H. *Non-surgical treatment of diseases of the glands and bones with a chapter on scrofula.* 170pp. 1894. London: James Epps.

145   Clarke, J.H. *The prescriber.* 382pp. 1983. Saffron Walden, Essex: Health Science Press. First published in 1885 in London.
The definitive prescriber, now in its 9th edition.

146   Clarke, J.H. *Radium as an internal remedy especially exemplified in cases of skin-disease and cancer.* 151pp. 1908. London: The Homoeopathic Publishing Co.

147   Clarke, J.H. *The revolution in medicine.* 88pp. 1886. London: Keene and Ashwell.

147A   Clarke, J.H. *Rheumatism and sciatica.* 189pp. 1892. London: James Epps.

148   Clarke, J.H. *Therapeutics of the serpent poisons.* 32pp. 1893. London: The Homoeopathic Publishing Co.
Materia medica essays of a very high standard.

149   Clarke, J.H. *Thomas Skinner, M.D. A biographical sketch.* 93pp. 1907. London: The Homoeopathic Publishing Co.

150   Clarke, J. H. *Whooping cough cured with coqueluchin its homoeopathic nosode.* 106pp. n.d. New Delhi, India: B. Jain. First published in 1906 in London.

151   Clarke, J.H. (editor). *Odium medicum and homoeopathy: 'The Times' correspondence.* 126pp. 1888. London: The Homoeopathic Publishing Co.
Dispute over the dismissal of a surgeon for co-operating with a homoeopath.

152   Close, Stuart. *Genius of homoeopathy.* 274pp. 1981. New Delhi, India: B. Jain. First published in 1924 in Philadelphia.
The most erudite essays on the philosophy of homoeopathy from the close of the 'American Golden Age'.

153   Clover, Anne. *Homoeopathy: a patient's guide.* 96pp. 1984. Wellingborough, Northamptonshire: Thorsons.
An introduction to homoeopathy.

154   Coats, Peter. *The homeopathic aide-memoire.* 96pp. 1980. Holsworthy, Devon: Health Science Press.
A simply written text.

155   Committee of Inquiry into Chiropractic, Osteopathy, Homoeopathy and Naturopathy. *Report of the Committee of Inquiry into chiropractic, osteopathy, homoeopathy and naturopathy.* 925pp. 1977. Canberra, Australia: Australian Government Publishing Service.

156   Committee on Pharmacopoeia of the American Institute of Homoeopathy. *The American Homoeopathic Pharmacopoeia.* 549pp. 1928. Philadelphia, Pennsylvania: Boericke and Tafel.

157   Cook, Trevor M. *Samuel Hahnemann: the founder of homoeopathic medicine.* 192pp. 1981. Wellingborough, Northamptonshire: Thorsons.
A popular biography.

158   Coulter, Harris L. *Divided legacy: the conflict between homoeopathy and the American Medical Association (Science and Ethics in American Medicine 1800–1914).* 568pp. 1982. Richmond, California: North Atlantic Books. Originally volume 3 of a three-volume history of American medicine.

159   Coulter, H.L. *Homoeopathic influences in 19th century allopathic therapeutics*. 86pp. 1977. St. Louis, Missouri: Formur.
A technical, historical and philosophical study.

160   Coulter, H.L. *Homoeopathic medicine*. 73pp. 1972. Washington, D.C.: American Foundation for Homoeopathy.
An introductory discussion.

161   Coulter, H.L. *Homoeopathic science and modern medicine, the physics of healing with microdoses*. 157pp. 1981. Richmond, California: North Atlantic Books.
Highly recommended.

162   Cowperthwaite, A.C. *Disorders of menstruation*. 73pp. 1981. New Delhi, India: B. Jain.
A useful handbook.

163   Cowperthwaite, A.C. *A textbook of gynaecology* 549pp. 1981. New Delhi, India: B. Jain. First published in 1888.
A very complete account of homoeopathic gynaecology.

164   Cowperthwaite, A.C. *A textbook of materia medica and therapeutics: characteristic, analytical and comparative*. 895pp. 1982. New Delhi, India: B. Jain.
One of the most valuable materia medicas. Recommended to all practitioners. Now into its 13th edition.

165   Cox, Donovan and T.W. Hyne-Jones. *Before the doctor comes ...* 32pp. n.d. Rustington, Sussex: Health Science Press.
A guide to dealing with minor ailments written by two businessmen.

166   Crews, Richard. *Introductory workbook in homeopathy*. 50pp. 1978. Berkeley, California: Homoeopathic Educational Services.
Highly recommended.

167   Curie, P.F. *Domestic practice of homoeopathy*. 302pp. 1850. London: W. Headland.

168   Curie, P.F. *Principles of homoeopathy*. 195pp. 1837. London: Thomas Hurst.

169   Curtis, J.T. and J. Lillie. *An epitome of homoeopathic practice*. 206pp. 1880. London: James Epps.

170   Dearborn, Frederick M. *American homoeopathy in the World War*. 447pp. 1923. Chicago, Illinois: The American Institute of Homoeopathy.

171   Derrick, Ken. *Medicine without fears*. 194pp. 1984. Bognor Regis, Sussex: New Horizon.
   An overview.

172   Dewey, W.A. *Essentials of homoeopathic materia medica and homoeopathic pharmacy*. 372pp. 1983. New Delhi, India: World Homoeopathic Links.
   A series of quizzes with answers, on the principles of homoeopathy, homoeopathic pharmacy and homoeopathic materia medica. Useful for students.

173   Dewey, W.A. *Essentials of homoeopathic therapeutics; being a quiz compend of the application of homoeopathic remedies to diseased states*. 290pp. 1981. New Delhi, India: B. Jain. First published in 1897.

174   Dewey, W.A. *Practical homoeopathic therapeutics*. 479pp. 1983. New Delhi, India: B. Jain. First published in 1934 in Philadelphia.
   Exclusively about homoeopathic prescribing.

175   Dhawale, M. L. *Principles and practice of homoeopathy*. 1983. Bombay, India: Homoeopathic Postgraduate Association.
   Highly recommended.

176   Drummond, John. *Popular guide to homoeopathy*. 364pp. 1890. London: Leath and Ross.

177   Dudgeon, R. E. *Hahnemann, the founder of scientific therapeutics*. 112pp. 1882. London: E. Gould.
   The Hahnemann Lecture of 1882.

178   Dudgeon, R.E. (collected and arranged by). *Hahnemann's therapeutic hints*. 59pp. 1894. London: E. Gould.

179   Dudgeon, R.E. *Lectures on the theory and practice of homoeopathy*. 565pp. 1982. New Delhi, India: B. Jain.
   Originally given as lectures at the Hahnemann Hospital in 1852–53.

180   Dudgeon, R.E. (editor). *Repertory of homoeopathic materia medica*. Volume 1: ch. 1–3, 287pp. Volume 2: ch. 4–15, 597pp. Ch. 18, A95pp.

Ch. 24, B145pp. No other chapters have been traced. 1878–85. Liverpool: Hahnemann Publishing Society. The most important British repertory, known colloquially as the 'Cypher repertory'. Issued in sections. Private bindings only.

181 Dudgeon, R.E. and J. Rutherford Russell (editors). *An introduction to the study of homoeopathy.* 253pp. 1865. London: J. Leath.

182 Dudgeon, R.E. and others. *Materia medica.* Volume 1: *Physiological and applied.* 726pp. 1884. London: Tubner and Co.

183 Duncan, Thomas C. *Children, acid and alkaline. The law of diet selection, contraria. The therapeutic law, similia.* 148pp. 1980. New Delhi, India: World Homoeopathic Links. First published in 1878 in Philadelphia.

184 Dunham, Carroll. *Homoeopathy the science of therapeutics: a collection of papers elucidating and illustrating the principles of homoeopathy.* 529pp. 1877. Philadelphia, Pennsylvania: Boericke and Tafel. Invaluable essays from a classical homoeopath.

185 Dunham, C. *Lectures on materia medica.* 446pp. 1982. New Delhi, India: World Homoeopathic Links.

186 Dunham, C. *Symptoms, their study: or, 'how to take the case'.* 24pp. n.d. New Delhi, India: Indian Books and Periodicals Syndicate.

187 Dunsford, Harris. *The pathogenic effects of some of the principal homoeopathic remedies.* 276pp. 1838. London: H. Baillière.

188 Dunsford, H. *The practical advantages of homoeopathy. Illustrated by numerous cases.* 215pp. London: H. Baillière.

189 Dutta, A.C. *Homoeopathic treatment systematised and simplified.* 216pp. 1981. New Delhi, India: B. Jain.

190 Dutta, A.C. *Homoeopathy in the light of modern science.* 136pp. 1983. New Delhi, India: B. Jain.

191 Epps, John. *Homoeopathy and its principles explained.* 320pp. 1801. London: W. and J. Piper.

192 Everest, Rev. Thomas R. *A popular view of homoeopathy.* 243pp. 1842. New York: William Radde.

193   Farrington, E.A. *Clinical materia medica.* 826pp. 1908. New Delhi, India: B. Jain. First published in Philadelphia.
One of the classical materia medica. Often used as a textbook in college courses.

194   Farrington, E.A. *Comparative materia medica.* 552pp. 1983. New Delhi, India: B. Jain.
Recommended. A scholarly materia medica to help understand remedies by comparison.

195   Farrington, E.A. *Lesser writings with therapeutic hints.* 407pp. 1982. New Delhi, India: B. Jain.
An erudite and useful collection of articles.

196   Farrington, Harvey. *Homoeopathy and homoeopathic prescribing.* 264pp. n.d. New Delhi, India: B. Jain.
An Indian reprint of a self-teaching text for graduate physicians arranged as forty-three lessons.

197   Finke, B. *On high potencies and homoeopathics. Clinical cases and observations.* 131pp. 1865. Philadelphia, Pennsylvania: A. J. Tafel, Homoeopathic Pharmacy.

198   Fisher, Charles E. *A handbook on the diseases of children and their homoeopathic treatment.* 1070pp. 1937. Calcutta, India: M. Bhattacharyya.

199   Fortier-Bernoville (translated by Raj Kumar Mukerji). *Diabetes mellitus.* 32pp. n.d. New Delhi, India: B. Jain.

200   Fortier-Bernoville (translated by R. K. Mukerji). *Syphilis and sycosis.* 133pp. n.d. New Delhi, India: B. Jain.

201   Fortier-Bernoville (translated by R.K. Mukerji). *Therapeutics of the diseases of liver and of biliary ducts.* 104pp. 1977. New Delhi, India: B. Jain.

202   Fortier-Bernoville (translated by R.K. Mukerji). *What we must not do in homoeopathy.* 74pp. 1974. New Delhi, India: B. Jain.

203   Fortier-Bernoville and L. A. Rousseau (translated by R.K. Mukerji). *Chronic rheumatism.* 58pp. 1982. New Delhi, India: B. Jain.

204   Fortier-Bernoville and L. A. Rousseau (translated by R.K.

Mukerji). *Remedies of circulatory and respiratory system.* 102pp. 1976. New Delhi, India: B. Jain.
A translation of lectures given in France.

205   Fortier-Bernoville and others (translated by R.K. Mukerji). *Eruptive fevers and contagious diseases of children.* 102pp. 1977. New Delhi, India: B. Jain.

206   Foubister, D.M. *The significance of past history in homoeopathic prescribing.* 11pp. 1962. London: The British Homoeopathic Association.
The well known 'never been well since' syndrome.

207   Frerleigh, M. *Homoeopathic practice of medicine: embracing the history, diagnosis and treatment of diseases in general, including those peculiar to females and the management of children.* 201pp. 1862. New York: Charles T. Hurlburt, Homoeopathic Pharmaceutist.

208   Gallavardin, *Doctor* (translated by I. Foulon). *The homoeopathic treatment of alcoholism.* 138pp. n.d. New Delhi, India: Jolly Enterprises. First published in 1890 in Philadelphia.
A fascinating insight into the history of French homoeopathy and pharmacy.

209   Gallavardin, Jean Pierre (translated by R.K. Mukerji). *Plastic medicine.* 24pp. n.d. New Delhi, India: World Homoeopathic Links.
A treatise on avoiding plastic surgery.

210   Gallavardin, J.P. (translated by R.K. Mukerji). *Psychism and homoeopathy.* 207pp. 1982. New Delhi, India: World Homoeopathic Links.
A great work of humane nineteenth-century homoeopathic psychiatry. Still of value.

211   Gallavardin, J.P. (translated by R.K. Mukerji). *Repertory and materia medica of psychic medicines.* 1982. New Delhi, India: World Homoeopathic Links.
A companion to *Psychism and homoeopathy.*

212   Gentry, William D. *Concordance repertory of the more characteristic symptoms of the materia medica.* 6 volumes. 1890. New York: Boericke and Tafel.
A very important work.

213   Gentry, W.D. *The rubrical and regional textbook of the homoeopathic materia medica with a section on the urine and urinary organs.* 239pp. 1983. New Delhi, India: World Homoeopathic Links. First published in 1890 in Philadelphia.

214   Ghosh, S.K. *Clinical experience with some rare nosodes.* 109pp. 1956. Calcutta, India: P.K. Bose.

215   Gibson, D.M. *Elements of homoeopathy.* 38pp. n.d. London: British Homoeopathic Association.
An introduction for doctors and medical students with an interest in homoeopathy.

216   Gibson, D.M. *First aid homoeopathy in accidents and ailments.* 84pp. 1978. London: British Homoeopathic Association.
A very clearly written guide.

217   Gibson, D.M. (edited by Marianne Harling and Brian Katlan). *Short materia medica of homoeopathic remedies.* 256pp. To be published in 1985. Beaconsfield, Buckinghamshire: Beaconsfield.

218   Gibson Miller, R. *Comparative value of symptoms in the selection of the remedy.* 24pp. n.d. New Delhi, India: B. Jain.
An invaluable reference book.

219   Gilchrist, J.G. *The homoeopathic treatment of surgical diseases.* 413pp. 1873. Chicago, Illinois: C.S. Halsey.

220   Gliddon, A.J.L. *Stepping stones to electro-homoeopathy (Count Mattei's system of medicine).* 295pp. 1930. London: Count Mattei's Remedies.
A book for the lay person to introduce this type of medicine.

221   Government of India, Ministry of Health. *Homoeopathic pharmacopoeia of India.* Volume 1: 277pp. 1974. Volume 2: 190pp. 1975. Volume 3: 155pp. 1978. New Delhi, India: The Controller of Publications, Government of India Press.

222   Granier, Michel (translated by H.E. Wilkinson and C.A.C. Clark). *Conférences upon homoeopathy.* 425pp. 1860. London: Leath and Ross.

223   Gregg, Rollin R. *Consumption: its cause and nature. To which is*

21

added, the therapeutics of tuberculous affections by H.C. Allen. 477pp. 1889. Ann Arbor, Michigan: Ann Arbor.

224   Grossinger, Richard. *Planet medicine: from stone age shamanism to post-industrial healing.* 436pp. 1982. Boulder, Colorado: Shambala Press.
A fascinating cross-cultural analysis.

225   Guernsey, Egbert. *Homoeopathic domestic medicine. With chapters on physiology, hygiene, anatomy and an abridged materia medica.* 649pp. 1858. New York: William Ryde.

226   Guernsey, Henry N. *The application of the principles and practice of homoeopathy to obstetrics and the disorders peculiar to women and young children.* 761pp. n.d. New Delhi, India: B. Jain. First published in 1875 in Philadelphia.
One of the most important works ever published on obstetrics in homoeopathy.

227   Guernsey, H.N. *Notes of lectures on materia medica delivered in the Hahnemann Medical College of Philadelphia.* 235pp. 1873. Philadelphia, Pennsylvania: William P. Kildare.

228   Guernsey, Joseph (editor). *Keynotes to the materia medica as taught by Henry N. Guernsey.* 263pp. 1939. Calcutta, India: Sett Dey.
Consists of a series of lectures delivered to students of the Hahnemann Medical School of Philadelphia in 1871–73.

229   Guernsey, William Jefferson. *Desires and aversions.* 35pp. n.d. New Delhi, India: Indian Books and Periodicals Syndicate. First published in *c.*1950.
A useful aide.

230   Guernsey, W.J. *The homoeopathic therapeutics of haemorrhoids.* 142pp. 1982. New Delhi, India: World Homoeopathic Links.
A comprehensive study.

231   Guernsey, W.J. *Menstruation.* 17pp. n.d. Calcutta, India: Salzer.

232   Gunavante, S.M. *Introduction to homoeopathic prescribing.* 303pp. 1982. New Delhi, India: World Homoeopathic Links.
A practical modern textbook for professional use.

22

233 Gupta, A.C. *Materia medica of bowel nosodes.* 42pp. 1982. New Delhi, India: Pratap.
An excellent textbook.

234 Gupta, B.P. *Encyclopaedia of homoeopathy.* 992pp. 1971. New Delhi, India: Homoeopathic Agency.
Includes a materia medica, repertory, etc.

235 Gutman, William. *Homoeopathy: the fundamentals of its philosophy and the essence of its remedies.* 158pp. 1978. Bombay, India: Homoeopathic Medical Publishers.
A classical exposition.

236 Gutman, W. *The little homoeopathic physician.* 41pp. 1961. Philadelphia, Pennsylvania: Boericke and Tafel.
Good.

237 Hael, Richard (translated by Marie L. Wheeler, edited by J.H. Clarke and F.J. Wheeler). *Samuel Hahnemann: his life and work.* 2 volumes 958pp. 1922. London: The Homoeopathic Publishing Co.
This is the definitive study of Hahnemann.

238 Hahnemann, Samuel (edited by Dudley Pemberton, annotated by R. Hughes). *The chronic diseases, their peculiar nature and their homoeopathic cure.* 2 volumes. 1620pp. 1981. New Delhi, India: B. Jain.
The most comprehensive homoeopathic text available. Translated from the 2nd edition of 1835 by Professor Louis Tafel.

239 Hahnemann, S. (translated by R.E. Dudgeon). *Hahnemann's defence of the organon of rational medicine and his previous homoeopathic works against the attacks of Professor Hecker. An explanatory commentary on the homoeopathic system.* 130pp. 1896. Philadelphia, Pennsylvania: Boericke and Tafel.

240 Hahnemann, S. (translated by R.E. Dudgeon). *The lesser writings.* 881pp. 1851. London: W. Headland.
An essential and principal work.

241 Hahnemann, S. (translated by R.E. Dudgeon). *Materia medica pura.* Volume 1: *Aconitum–ipecacuanha.* 718pp. Volume 2: *Ledum–verbuscum.* 708pp. 1983. New Delhi, India: B. Jain. First published in 1880 in London.
The original provings.

23

242   Hahnemann, S. *The organon of medicine.* The original work on homoeopathic medicine, available in several translations, for example: (i) R.E. Dudgeon. (5th edition). 224pp. 1982. New Delhi, India: B. Jain. (ii) William Boericke. (6th edition). 314pp. 1983. New Delhi, India: B. Jain. First published in 1935 in Philadelphia. (iii) The modern translation of J. Kunzli, A. Naude and P. Pendleton. (6th edition). 270pp. 1983. London: Victor Gollancz.

243   Hale, Edwin M. *Lectures on diseases of the heart with a materia medica of the new heart remedies* (and a repertory of heart symptoms compiled by E.R. Snader). 478pp. 1980. New Delhi, India: B. Jain. Second edition published in 1875.

244   Hale, R. Douglas. *Eight lectures on the homoeopathic treatment of acute and chronic bronchitis, laryngitis, pleuritis, pneumonia, phthisis, pulmonalis and pericarditis.* 95pp. 1877. London: Henry Turner.

245   Halsey, C.S. and Geo. E. Halsey. *Halsey's homoeopathic guide. For families, travellers, missionaries, pioneers, miners etc.* 262pp. 1885. Chicago, Illinois: C.S. and Geo.E. Halsey.

246   Hamilton. *The flora homoeopathica: illustrations and descriptions of the medicinal plants used as homoeopathic remedies.* 2 volumes. 1852. Reprinted in facsimile, 1 volume: 523pp. 1981. London: Faculty of Homoeopathy.
A historical curiosity.

247   Hamlyn, Edward (editor). *The healing art of homoeopathy: the organon of Samuel Hahnemann.* 110pp. 1979. Beaconsfield, Buckinghamshire: Beaconsfield.
An abbreviated version of the organon, meant as an aide to practitioners.

248   Hands, Joseph. *Homoeopathy and other modern systems contrasted with allopathy. Also a treatise on diets and digestion.* 426pp. n.d. London: Leath and Ross.

249   Hansen, Oscar. *A textbook of materia medica and therapeutics of rare homoeopathic remedies.* 121pp. n.d. New Delhi, India: B. Jain. First published in 1899.
This was designed as a supplement to Dr. Cowperthwaite's materia medica.

250   Hatteria, Homee A.S. *Organon of esoteric principles of homoeotherapeutics.* 167pp. 1957. Name of publisher not given.

251 Heinigke, Carl. *Pathogenic outlines of homoeopathic drugs.* 576pp. 1880. Philadelphia, Pennsylvania: Boericke and Tafel.

252 Hempel, Charles J. *Homoeopathy, a principle in nature, its scientific universality unfolded; its development and philosophy explained, and its applicability to the treatment of disease shown by Charles J. Hempel.* 248pp. 1860. Philadelphia, Pennsylvania: William Radde.

253 Hempel, C.J. *Organon of specific homoeopathy; or, an inductive exposition of the principles of the homoeopathic healing art addressed to physicians and intelligent laymen.* 212pp. 1854, Philadelphia, Pennsylvania: Rademacher and Sheek.

254 Hempel, C.J. and Jacob Beakley. *Manual of homoeopathic theory and practice with an elementary treatise on the homoeopathic treatment of surgical diseases.* 1076pp. 1859. Philadelphia, Pennsylvania: William Radde.

255 Henderson, William. *Homoeopathy fairly represented in reply to Dr. Simpson's '"Homoeopathy" misrepresented'.* 276pp. 1853. Edinburgh: Thomas Constable and Co.

256 Henderson, W. *An inquiry into the homoeopathic practice of medicine.* 238pp. 1865. London: J. Leath.

257 Henriques, A. *The homoeopathic medical dictionary and home guide.* 261pp. n.d. London: W. Headland.

258 Henshaw, George Russell. *A scientific approach to homoeopathy.* 213pp. 1980. Hicksville, New York: Exposition Press.
Papers from medical journals that cover different aspects of homoeopathy.

259 Hering, Constantine (revised and enlarged by E.A. Farrington). *Condensed materia medica.* 1086pp. 1983. New Delhi, India: B. Jain. A reprint of the 3rd edition of 1884.

260 Hering, C. *Guiding symptoms of the materia medica.* 10 volumes, each over 500pp. 1984. New Delhi, India: B. Jain. First published in 1880 by the American Homoeopathic Publishing Co.
One of the most valuable of all homoeopathic books to practitioners.

261 Hering, C. *The homoeopathic domestic physician.* 458pp. 1883. New Delhi, India: B. Jain.
An important work. The first-ever book for domestic use.

25

262   Hering, C. (editor). *Dr. H. Gross' comparative materia medica.*
520pp. n.d. New Delhi, India: B. Jain.
Each remedy described is surveyed very fully.

263   Hill, B. L. *The homoeopathic practice of surgery together with operative surgery.* 223pp. 1855. Cleveland, Ohio: J.B. Cobb and Company.

264   Hobhouse, Rosa Waugh. *Life of Christian Samuel Hahnemann founder of homoeopathy.* 288pp. 1933. London: C.W. Daniel.
A thorough biography.

265   Holcombe, William H. *The scientific basis of homoeopathy.* 304pp. 1852. Cincinnati, Ohio: H.W. Derby and Co. Publishers.

266   Homoeopathic Development Foundation (compiled by). *Homoeopathy for the family.* 36pp. 1983. London: Homoeopathic Development Foundation.
An introductory guide.

267   Homoeopathic Publishing Company. *Doctor Lowe's sacrifice, or, the triumph of homoeopathy.* 96pp. 1975. London: The Homoeopathic Publishing Company.

268   Hoyme, Temple. *Clinical therapeutics.* Volume 1: 602pp. 1878. Chicago, Illinois: Duncan Brothers, Printers. Volume 2: 643pp. 1880. Chicago, Illinois: Culver, Page and Hoyne and Co., Printers.

269   Hubbard-Wright, Elizabeth. *A brief study course in homoeopathy.* 102pp. 1983. St. Louis, Missouri: Formur.
A concisely written introduction to the methodology of homoeopathic science.

270   Hughes, Richard. *Hahnemann as a medical philosopher: the organon.* 92pp. 1882. London: E. Gould.
Given as the 2nd Hahnemann Lecture (1881).

271   Hughes, R. *Knowledge of the physician. A course of lectures, delivered at the Boston University School of medicine, May 1884.* 292pp. 1980. New Delhi, India: World Homoeopathic Links. First published in 1884.
A well written and scholarly account of a course of twelve lectures delivered in Boston by this English homoeopath.

272 Hughes, R. *A manual of pharmacodynamics.* 962pp. 1983. New Delhi, India: B. Jain. This 6th edition was first published in 1893 in London.
A scholarly reference materia medica.

273 Hughes, R. *A manual of therapeutics, according to the method of Hahnemann.* Part I: *General diseases—diseases of the nervous system.* 444pp. 1877. Part II: 449pp. 1878. London: Leath and Ross.

274 Hughes, R. *Principles and practice of homoeopathy.* 795pp. 1983. New Delhi, India: World Homoeopathic Links. First published in 1878 in London.
A work of rigorous scholarship. Recommended.

275 Hughes, R. and J.P. Dake (editors). *A cyclopaedia of drug pathogenesy.* 4 volumes + repertory. 1979. New Delhi, India: World Homoeopathic Links. First published in 1886 in London.
An outstanding work, issued under the auspices of the British Homoeopathic Society and the American Institute of Homoeopathy.

276 Irish Homoeopathic Society. *A concise view of the system of homoeopathy and refutation of the objections.* 240pp. 1848. Dublin: James McGlashan.

277 Iyer, T.S. *Beginners guide to homoeopathy.* 543pp. 1984. New Delhi, India: B. Jain.
Written by a layman in 1948 and still widely used by students.

278 Jahr, G.H.G. (translated by Charles J. Hempel). *The clinical guide or pocket repertory for the treatment of acute and chronic diseases.* 624pp. 1891. Philadelphia, Pennsylvania: Hahnemann Publishing House.

279 Jahr, G.H.G. (translated by C.J. Hempel). *Diseases of females and infants at the breast.* 346pp. n.d. New Delhi, India: B. Jain. First published in 1856 in New York.

280 Jahr, G.H.G. *Family practice or simple directions in homoeopathic domestic medicine.* 276pp. 1982. New Delhi, India: B. Jain.
A discussion of the remedies that can most usefully be applied in the home.

281 Jahr, G.H.G. *Jahr's new manual of the homoeopathic materia medica with Possart's additions, with reference to well authenticated observations at the*

27

sick bed and accompanied by an alphabetical repertory. 924pp. 1859. New York: William Radde.

282   Jahr, G.H.G. (translated by P.F. Currie). *Manual of homoeopathic medicine.* Volume 1: 631pp. Volume 2: 620pp. 1878. London: H. Baillière.

283   Jahr, G.H.G. (translated by Charles J. Hempel). *Therapeutic guide: the most important results of more than forty years' practice.* 364pp. 1980. New Delhi, India: B. Jain. First published in 1869 in Philadelphia.
Jahr's finest work and still a valuable text for practitioners.

284   Johnson, I.D. *A guide to homoeopathic practice designed for the use of families and private individuals.* 494pp. 1883. Philadelphia, Pennsylvania: F.E. Boericke.

285   Joslin, B.F. *Principles of homoeopathy. A series of lectures.* 185pp. 1850. New York: William Ryde.

286   Jouanny, Jacques. *The essentials of homoeopathic materia medica.* 454pp. 1980. Lyon, France: Laboratoires Boiron.

287   Jouanny, J. *The essentials of homoeopathic therapeutics.* 418pp. 1980. Lyon, France: Laboratoires Boiron.
Details the French approach to homoeopathy. Good on skin conditions.

288   Julian, O.A. (translated by V. Munday). *Materia medica of new homoeopathic remedies* 637pp. 1979. Beaconsfield, Buckinghamshire: Beaconsfield.
A rich collection of over one hundred new remedies.

289   Julian, O.A. (translated by R. Mulserji). *Treatise on dynamised micro immuno-therapy, biotherapies and nosodes (part 1: 161pp). Practical materia medica of biotherapies and nosodes* (part 2: 549pp). 1980. New Delhi, India: B. Jain.
A collection of theory, historical vignettes and materia medica.

290   Kaufman, Martin. *Homoeopathy in America: the rise and fall of a medical heresy.* 205pp. 1971. Baltimore, Maryland: Johns Hopkins University Press.

291   Kent, James Tyler (revised, corrected and augmented by

Pierre Schmidt and Diwan Harish Chand). *Kent's Final general repertory of the homoeopathic materia medica.* 1423pp. 1982. New Delhi, India: National Homoeopathic Pharmacy.

292   Kent, J.T. *Lectures on homoeopathic materia medica with new remedies.* 1107pp. n.d. New Delhi, India: Homoeopathic Publications. First published in 1904 in Philadelphia.
A principal work.

293   Kent, J.T. *Lectures on homoeopathic philosophy.* 267pp. 1983. New Delhi, India: B. Jain. First published in 1900 in Philadelphia.
Highly recommended. The principal work in the classical Hahnemannian tradition.

294   Kent, J.T. *New remedies: clinical cases, lesser writings, aphorisms and precepts.* 698pp. 1981. New Delhi, India: B. Jain. First published in 1926 in Chicago.
Another important work: reports of Kent's work by other hands.

295   Kent, J.T. *Repertory of the homoeopathic materia medica.* 1532pp. 1983. New Delhi, India: World Homoeopathic Links.
The best and most comprehensive repertory. This edition includes a section by Margaret Tyler and John Weir on how to study and use the repertory.

296   Kent, J.T. *What the doctor needs to know in order to make a successful prescription.* 56pp. 1980 New Delhi, India: B. Jain.
Recommended.

297   Kichlu, K.L. and L.R.N. Bose. *A text book of descriptive medicine with clinical methods and homoeopathic therapeutics.* 1049pp. 1982. New Delhi, India: B. Jain.
An Indian medical text for students studying medicine in homoeopathic schools in India.

298   Kidd, Joseph. *The law of therapeutics, or, the science and art of medicine. A sketch.* 232pp. 1878. London: C. Kegan Paul and Co.

299   King, William Harvey. *History of homoeopathy and its institutions in America.* 4 volumes. 1905. New York: The Lewis Publishing Company.

300   Klunker, W. *Synthetic repertory.* Volume 3: *Sleep, dreams and sexuality.* 587pp. 1974. Heidelberg, W. Germany: Karl F. Haug.
Rubrics in English, French and German.

29

Contains three separate indices, separately paged. This work has been derived from about sixteen other repertories and is thoroughly cross-referenced.

301   Knerr, Calvin B. *Drug relationship.* 223pp. 1971. Calcutta, India: Aggrawal. First published in 1936.
Extracts from Knerr's repertory.

302   Knerr, C.B. *Repertory of Hering's guiding symptoms of our materia medica.* 1232pp. 1982. New Delhi, India: B. Jain.
A useful aid to understanding Hering's work.

303   Langbridge, R.H. (compiler). ABC of homoeopathy. An anthology of homoeopathic teaching. 109pp. n.d. London: The Homoeopathic Publishing Co.

304   Laurie, Joseph. *The homoeopathic domestic medicine.* 1082pp. 1885. London: Leath and Ross.

305   Lee, Edmund J. (editor). *Repertory of the characteristic symptoms, clinical and pathogenic, of the homoeopathic materia medica.* 163pp. 1889. Philadelphia, Pennsylvania: Name of publisher not given. Published as a supplement to *The homoeopathic physician.*

306   Leeser, Otto (translated by Linn J. Boyd). *Textbook of homeopathic materia medica: inorganic medicinal substances.* 1003pp. 1980. New Delhi, India: B. Jain. First published in 1932 in Philadelphia.
A comprehensive account of all ten remedies from mineral sources.

307   Leeser, O. *Textbook of homoeopathy.* 5 volumes + index. Heidelberg, W. Germany: Karl F. Haug. 2nd edition in progress.

308   Lessell, Colin B. *Homoeopathy for physicians: a practical introduction to prescribing.* 160pp. 1983. Wellingborough, Northamptonshire: Thorsons.

309   Lilienthal, Samuel. *Homeopathic therapeutics.* 1154pp. 1983. New Delhi, India: B. Jain. 3rd edition published in 1890 in Philadelphia.
Generally considered the most complete guide to therapeutics available.

310   Lippe, A.D. *Text book of materia medica.* 716pp. 1981. New Delhi, India: B. Jain. First published in 1865.

Originally prepared for students at the Homoeopathic Medical College of Pennsylvania.

311   Lippe, Adolph von. *Key notes of the homoeopathic materia medica.* 163pp. 1980. New Delhi, India: B. Jain.
Intended as a supplement to the major works.

312   Lippe, A. von. *Key notes and red line symptoms of the materia medica.* 275pp. 1982. New Delhi, India: World Homoeopathic Links.
A handy quick-reference book.

313   Lippe, Constantine. *Repertory to the more characteristic symptoms of the materia medica.* 438pp. 1949. Calcutta, India: M. Bhattacharyya.
First published in 1879 in New York.
An exhaustive, professional study.

314   Livingston, R. *Homoeopathy—born 1810—and still going strong.* 67pp. 1973. London: Asher Asher Press.

315   Livingston, R. *Homoeopathy: the power to heal.* 24pp. 1976. Poole, Dorset: Asher Asher Press.

316   Lutze, F.H. *Duration of action and antidotes of the principal homoeopathic remedies with their complementary and inimical relations.* 48pp. n.d. Lahore, Pakistan: Homoeopathic Stores and Hospital.

317   McGavack, Thomas Hodge. *The homoeopathic principle in therapeutics.* 204pp. 1932. Philadelphia, Pennsylvania: Boericke and Tafel.

318   MacKenzie, Frazer. *Homoeopathy. A live explanation of what homoeopathy is and what it means to your health.* 96pp. n.d. London: The Homoeopathic Publishing Co.
For the layman.

319   Malcom, John Gilmore and Oscar Burton Moss. *A regional and comparative materia medica.* 919pp. 1895. Chicago, Illinois: Malcolm and Moss Publishers.

320   Marcey, E.E. and F.W. Hunt. *The homoeopathic theory and practice of medicine.* Volume 1: 944pp. 1865. Volume 2: 952pp. 1865. New York: William Radde.

321   Marcey, E.E., J.C. Peters and Otto Fullgraff. *The elements of a new materia medica and therapeutics: based upon an entirely new collection of*

drug-provings and clinical experience. 767pp. n.d. Name of publisher not given.

322   Massy, R. Tuthill. *Mild medicine in contradistinction to severe medicine.* 117pp. 1859. London: Thomas Sanderson.

323   Matheson, Duncan. *On some of the diseases of women, their pathology and homoeopathic treatment: being four lectures delivered at the London Homoeopathic Hospital.* 76pp. 1876. London: Leath and Ross.

324   Mathur, K.N. *Diabetes mellitus: its diagnosis and treatment.* 75pp. 1982. New Delhi, India: B. Jain.

325   Mathur, K.N. *Guide to organon.* 148pp. 1982. New Delhi, India: B. Jain.
A question-and-answer guide to homoeopathic medicine.

326   Mathur, K.N. *Principles of prescribing: collected from clinical experiences of pioneers of homoeopathy.* 671pp. 1981. New Delhi, India: B. Jain.
A comprehensive volume.

327   Mathur, K.N. *Systematic materia medica of homoeopathic remedies with totality of characteristic symptoms, comparisons and various indications of each remedy.* 1068pp. 1982. New Delhi, India: B. Jain.
Recommended.

328   Maurey, E.A. (translated by Mark Clements). *A concise guide to homoeopathy.* 64pp. 1956. Hindhead, Surrey: Health Science Press.

329   Maurey, E.A. *Drainage in homoeopathy (detoxification).* 60pp. 1982. Rustington, Sussex: Health Science Press.
A work for practitioners on a controversial practice.

330   Maurey, E.A. (translated by Geoffrey A. Dudley). *Homoeopathic practice in thirty remedies: rapid treatment for common ailments.* 95pp. 1981. Wellingborough, Northamptonshire: Thorsons.

331   Maurey, E.A. *Homoeopathic treatment of children's ailments: remedies for common ailments.* 94pp. 1982. Wellingborough, Northamptonshire: Thorsons.
A clear practical manual.

332   Miller, R. Gibson. *Dr. R. Gibson Miller's Relationship of remedies.* 43pp. n.d. London: The Homoeopathic Publishing Co.
Remedies are arranged alphabetically.

333   Mitchell, G. Ruthven. *Homoeopathy.* 200pp. 1975. London: W.H. Allen.

334   Moffat, John L. *Homoeopathic therapeutics on ophthalmology.* 166pp. 1916. Philadelphia, Pennsylvania: Boericke and Tafel.

335   Monroe, A.L. *Method of memorising the materia medica.* 50pp. 1980. New Delhi, India: World Homoeopathic Links.

336   Moore, George L. *Popular guide to homoeopathy, for families and private use.* 158pp. 1858. Manchester: Henry Turner.

337   Morgan, Samuel. *The textbook for domestic practice, being plain and concise directions for the administration of homoeopathic medicines in simple ailments.* 199pp. 1863. Bath, Avon: Edmund Capper.

338   Moskowitz, Richard. *Homoeopathic reasoning.* 17pp. 1980. Privately published by author.
Recommended.

339   Mukerji, Raj Kumar (compiler and translator). *Constitution and temperament.* 157pp. 1976. New Delhi, India: B. Jain.
French journal articles.

340   Mure, B. (arranged by Charles J. Hempel). *Dr. B. Mure's materia medica, or, provings of the principal animal and vegetable poisons of the Brazilian empire, and their application in the treatment of disease.* 218pp. 1854. New York: William Radde.

341   Muzumdar, K.P. *Pharmaceutical science in homoeopathy and pharmacodynamics.* 182pp. 1980. New Delhi, India: B. Jain.
A detailed study.

342   Nash, E.B. *How to take the case and find the similium.* 24pp. n.d. New Delhi, India: B. Jain.
An excellent pamphlet on the homoeopathic interview.

343   Nash, E.B. *Leaders for the use of sulphur with comparisons.* 80pp. 1981. New Delhi, India: World Homoeopathic Links. First published in 1898 in Philadelphia.
Insights into one of the most complex remedies.

33

344   Nash, E.B. *Leaders in homoeopathic therapeutics.* 516pp. 1983. New Delhi, India: B. Jain. First published in 1926 in Philadelphia.
An in-depth description of the main remedies including a useful grouping of types of remedy and classification according to use.

345   Nash, E.B. *Leaders in respiratory organs.* 168pp. 1962. Calcutta, India: Sett Dey. First published in 1909 in Philadelphia.

346   Nash, E.B. *Regional leaders.* 148pp. 1950. Calcutta, India: Sett Dey. First published in 1900 in Philadelphia.
A summary of the most important remedies for all the body and for a variety of ailments and conditions.

347   Nash, E.B. (collected by C. S. Sandhu). *Science of symptomatology and how shall we teach materia medica and therapeutics.* 39pp. 1981. New Delhi, India: National Homoeopathic Publishers.

348   Nash, E.B. *Testimony of the clinic.* 104pp. 1981. Calcutta, India: C. Ringer. First published in 1911 in Philadelphia.
Unique case studies from a master prescriber.

349   Neatby, Edwin Awdas and T.G. Stonham. *An index of aggravations and ameliorations.* 110pp. 1981. New Delhi, India: B. Jain. First published in 1927 in London.
A quick reference book.

350   Neatby, E.A. and T.G. Stonham. *A manual of homoeo-therapeutics.* 1048pp. 1927. London: J. Bale and Co. (Volume 2 of Bale's *Medical manuals for missionaries.*)

351   Neatby, T. Miller. *Homoeopathy reasoned out: a survey of the very latest medical and surgical methods of treatment proving incontestably the value of homoeopathy.* 31pp. n.d. London: The Homoeopathic Publishing Co.

352   Neidhard, C. *Pathogenetic and clinical repertory of the most prominent symptoms of the head with their concomitants and conditions.* 188pp. n.d. New Delhi, India: B. Jain.
Based on Allen's *Encyclopedia of materia medica.*

353   Niederkorn, Joseph S. *A handy reference book.* 156pp. 1925. Calcutta, India: Aggrawal.
An authoritative account.

354   Norton, A.B. *Ophthalmic diseases and therapeutics.* 659pp. 1978. New Delhi, India: B. Jain. First published in 1901 in Philadelphia.

355   Ortega, Procesco Sancez. *Notes on the miasms: Hahnemann's chronic diseases.* 295pp. 1980. New Delhi, India: Pratap.

356   Panos, Maesimund and Jane Heimlich. *Homoeopathic medicine at home.* 304pp. 1982. London: Corgi.

357   Patel, Ramanlal P. *The art of case taking and practical repertorisation.* 76pp. 1982. Kottayam, Kerala, India: Hahnemann Homoeopathic Pharmacy.
An immensely practical book.

358   Patel, R.P. *My experiments with fifty millesimal scale potencies according to the 6th edition of 'Organon of medicine'.* 137pp. 1960. Kottayam Kerala, India: Hahnemann Homoeopathic Pharmacy.

359   Patel, R.P. *What is tautopathy?* 108pp. 1981. Kottyam, Kerala, India: Hahnemann Homoeopathic Pharmacy.
A homoeopathic method of curing the side-effects of drugs.

360   Patel, R.P. and P. Elias. *A treatise on homoeopathic surgery.* 136pp. n.d. Kottayam, Kerala, India: Sai Homoeopathic Book Corporation.

361   Perry, Edward L. *Luyties' homoeopathic practice. The safe system to health for the entire family.* 160pp. 1977. St. Louis, Missouri: Formur.
Easy to read. For the layman.

362   Phatak, S.R. *A concise repertory of homoeopathic medicines.* 410pp. 1982. Bombay, India: The Homoeopathic Medical Publishers.

363   Phatak, S.R. *Materia medica of homoeopathic remedies.* 631pp. 1982. New Delhi, India: Indian Books and Periodical Syndicate.

364   Poirer, Jean (translated by R.K. Mukerjee). *Homoeopathic treatment of diseases of the heart.* 95pp. 1982. New Delhi, India: World Homoeopathic Links.

365   Pope, Alfred C. *Homoeopathy popularly explained, in reply to Mr. Dix's pamphlet, entitled 'Homoeopathy popularly exposed'.* Pages not numbered. 1854. London: Aylott and Co.

366   Pratt, Noel. *Homoeopathic prescribing.* 79pp. 1980. Beaconsfield, Buckinghamshire: Beaconsfield.

Pathological homoeopathy for students with an allopathic background. A new edition is due in January 1985.

367   Puddephatt, Noel. *The homoeopathic materia medica. How it should be used.* 32pp. 1972. Rustington, Sussex: Health Science Press. First published in 1945.

368   Puddephatt, N. *How to find the correct remedy. The values of symptoms and modalities peculiar to the patient.* 31pp. 1972. Rustington, Sussex: Health Science Press.

369   Puddephatt, N. *Puddephatt's primers.* 65pp. 1982. Saffron Walden, Essex: Health Science Press.
A good introduction for the student of homoeopathy.

370   Puddephatt, N. and Marjorie Kincaid-Smith. *Signposts to the homoeopathic remedies.* 132pp. *c*1978. Rustington, Sussex: Health Science Press.
Recommended.

371   Puhlmann, C.G. (translated by J. Foster). *Handbook of homoeopathic practice. Instructions for the clinical examination of the sick and their treatment according to homoeopathic principles with complete dietary and special reference to tropical diseases.* 609pp. 1897. Leipzig, Germany: Dr. Willmar Schwabe.

372   Pulford, Alfred T. and Dayton Turner Pulford. *Homoeopathic leaders in pneumonia.* 100pp. 1928. Toledo, Ohio: By authors.
An important work.

373   Pulford, A.T. and D.T. Pulford. *Homoeopathic materia medica, or graphic drug pictures and clinical comments.* 318pp. 1944. Toledo, Ohio: By authors.

374   Pulford, A.T. and D.T. Pulford. *Key to the homoeopathic materia medica.* 136pp. 1936. Toledo, Ohio: By authors.

375   Pulte, J.H. *The homoeopathic domestic medicine; containing the treatment of diseases, with popular explanations of anatomy, physiology, hygiene, hydropathy and domestic surgery.* 722pp. n.d. London: James Epps.

376   Quay, G.H. *A monograph of diseases of the nose and throat.* 207pp. 1969. Calcutta, India: Sett Dey.

377   Ramseyer, A.A. (translator and editor). *Rademacher's universal*

organ remedies. 104pp. 1980. New Delhi, India: World Homoeopathic Links. First published in 1909.

378   Rau, Gottlieb Ludwig (translated by Charles Julius Hempel). *Organon of the specific healing art.* 200pp. 1847. New York: William Ryde.

379   Raue, C. Sigmund. *Diseases of children: a textbook for the use of students and practitioners of medicine.* 776pp. 1979. New Delhi, India: B. Jain. First published in 1906.

380   Raue, C.S. *Special pathology and therapeutic hints.* 1039pp. n.d. New Delhi, India: B. Jain. A reprint from the 4th edition of 1896, published in Philadelphia.

381   Reith, Archibald. *Homoeopathy: its nature and relative value.* With an appendix by Dr. Dyce Brown. 56pp. 1868. Aberdeen: D. Wyllie and Son.

382   Roberts, Herbert A. *The principles and art of cure by homoeopathy: a modern textbook.* 285pp. 1976. Saffron Walden, Essex: Health Science Press. First published in 1936 in London.
A well written basic text for the beginning student.

383   Roberts, H.A. *The principles and practicability of Boenninghausen's therapeutic pocket book.* 76pp. 1935. Philadelphia, Pennsylvania: Boericke and Tafel.

384   Roberts, H.A. *'Sensations as if—'. A repertory of subjective symptoms.* 519pp. 1983. New Delhi, India: B. Jain. First published in 1937 in Philadelphia.
A comprehensive work.

385   Roberts, H.A. *The study of remedies by comparison.* 87pp. 1973. New Delhi, India: B. Jain.
One of the better guides for comparison, especially of the mental systems.

386   Ross, A.C. Gordon. *The amazing healer: arnica, and a dozen other homoeopathic remedies for aches, pains and strains.* 96pp. 1981. Wellingborough, Northamptonshire: Thorsons.

387   Ross, A.C.G. *Homoeopathic green medicine: a comparison between the homoeopathic and allopathic approaches to the healing powers in plants, weeds*

and trees. 96pp. 1981. Wellingborough, Northamptonshire: Thorsons.

388   Ross, A.C.G. *Homoeopathy: an introductory guide.* 64pp. 1982. Wellingborough, Northamptonshire: Thorsons.
Suited to lay enquirers.

389   Rousseau, L. and Fortier-Bernoville. *Diseases of the respiratory and digestive system of children.* 66pp. 1976. New Delhi, India: B. Jain.

390   Roy, C. *Etiology in homoeopathy.* 308pp. n.d. Calcutta, India: By author.

391   Royal, George. *A handy book of reference for students and general practitioners of homoeopathy.* 323pp. 1930. Philadelphia, Pennsylvania: Boericke and Tafel.

392   Royal, G. *Homoeopathic therapy of diseases of the brain and nerves.* 360pp. 1981. New Delhi, India: B. Jain. First published in c1923.

393   Royal, G. *Textbook of homoeopathic materia medica.* 404pp. 1920. Calcutta, India: Roysingh. First published in Philadelphia.
A very clear discussion.

394   Royal, G. *Text-book of homoeopathic theory and practice of medicine.* 689pp. 1980. New Delhi, India: B. Jain. First published in 1923 in Philadelphia.
A very comprehensive text for the practitioner.

395   Ruddock, Edward Harris (revised by T.M. Neatby). *The common diseases of infants and children.* 168pp. 1981. New Delhi, India: B. Jain. 6th edition was originally published in 1899.
A useful though dated book for mothers.

396   Ruddock, E.H. *The common diseases of women including the homoeopathic and general treatment of ailments peculiar to different periods of life.* 167pp. 1981. New Delhi, India: B. Jain. First published c.1930 in London.
One of the most widely used books on this subject.

397   Ruddock, E. H. *On consumption and tuberculosis of the lungs.* 126pp. 1873. London: The Homoeopathic Publishing Co.

398   Ruddock, E.H. *The lady's manual of homeopathic treatment in the*

various derangements incident to her sex. 279pp. 1974. Calcutta, India: M. Bhattacharyya. First published in 1866.

399   Ruddock, E.H. (revised by J.H. Clarke). *Ruddock's Homoeopathic vade maecum.* 922pp. n.d. New Delhi, India: Ashoka Publishing. First published in 1925 in London.
   Written for the layman.

400   Ruddock, E.H. *The stepping-stone to homoeopathy and health with clinical directory.* 366pp. 1981. New Delhi, India: B. Jain. First published in 1880 in London.
   An excellent basic treatise, geared towards the layman.

401   Ruddock, E.H. *Textbook of modern medicine and surgery on homoeopathic principles.* 1029pp. 1878. London: The Homoeopathic Publishing Co.

402   Russell, J. Rutherfurd (editor). *Homoeopathy in 1851.* 416pp. 1852. Edinburgh: James Hogg.

403   Salzer, L. (revised by N.K. Banerjee). *A repertory of the peculiar symptoms based on periodic drug disorders.* 96pp. 1980. New Delhi, India: World Homoeopathic Links.

404   Sampson, Marmaduke B. *Homoeopathy: its principles, theory and practice.* 204pp. 1866. London: Samuel Highley.

405   Sampson, M.B. *Truths and their reception, considered in relation to the doctrine of homoeopathy, to which are added various essays on the principles and statistics of homoeopathic practice.* 251pp. 1869. London: Samuel Highley.

406   Sankaran, P. *Indications and use of bowel nosodes.* 14pp. 1973. Bombay, India: Homoeopathic Medical Publishers.
   A comprehensive pamphlet.

407   Sankaran, P. *Some cross references to Kent's 'Repertory'.* 65pp. 1977. Bombay, India: Homoeopathic Medical Publishers.

408   Sankaran, P. *Some new provings.* 41pp. n.d. Bombay, India: Homoeopathic Medical Publishers.

409   Sankaran, P. *Some recent research and advances in homoeopathy.* 82pp. 1978. Bombay, India: Homoeopathic Medical Publishers.
   A review of scientific research since 1900.

410   Sankaran, P. *When the indicated remedies fail.* 20pp. 1976. Bombay, India: Homoeopathic Medical Publishers.

411   Santwani, M.T. *Common ailments of children and their homoeopathic management.* 480pp. 1983. New Delhi, India: B. Jain.
Recommended. Some twenty-six ailments are covered, together with the different children's constitutional types.

412   Santwani, M.T. *Deficiency diseases and their homoeopathic management.* 142pp. 1979. New Delhi, India: B. Jain.

413   Santwani, M.T. *Pain: types, significance and homoeopathic management.* 88pp. 1982. New Delhi, India: B. Jain.

414   Santwani, M.T. *Practical diet guide in homoeopathy; foods to be temporarily avoided during homoeopathic treatment.* 29pp. 1983. New Delhi, India: B. Jain.

415   Sarker, B.K. *Clinical relationships of drugs with their modalities.* 187pp. 1971. Calcutta, India: Roysingh.
A thorough compilation.

416   Sarker, B.K. *Essays on homoeopathy.* 1968. Calcutta, India: Hahnemann Publishing Co. (Ptc).

417   Sarker, B.K. (editor). *Up-to-date with nosodes.* 191pp. 1964. Calcutta, India: Roy Publishing Co.

418   Schmidt, Pierre. *The art of case taking.* 52pp. 1976. Bombay, India: Homoeopathic Medical Publishers.

419   Schmidt, Pierre. *Defective illnesses.* 73pp. 1980. Calcutta, India: Hahnemann Publishing Co. (Ptc). Reprinted from *Homoeotherapy*, 1974.

420   Scott, Keith A. and Linda A. McCourt. *Homoeopathy: the potent force of the minimum dose.* 128pp. 1982. Wellingborough, Northamptonshire: Thorsons.
An introductory review.

421 Sengupta, S. N. *The science and philosophy of homoeopathy (an elementary lesson)*. 164pp. 1931. Privately published by the author.

422 Shadman, Alonzo. *Who is your doctor and why*. 446pp. 1980. New Canaan, Connecticut: Keats.
   Highly recommended. One of the few comprehensive books on homoeopathy written for the general reader in non-technical terms.

423 Sharma, C.H. *A manual of homoeopathy and natural medicine*. 154pp. 1983. Wellingborough, Northamptonshire: Turnstone.
   An introduction.

424 Sharp, William. *An investigation of homoeopathy*. 347pp. 1856. London: Groombridge and Sons.

425 Sharp, W. *Tracts on homoeopathy*. Pages not numbered. 1859. London: Aylott and Co.

426 Shepherd, Dorothy. *Homoeopathy for the first-aider*. 72pp. 1982. Saffron Walden, Essex: Health Science press. First published in 1945.
   Recommended.

427 Shepherd, D. *Homeopathy in epidemic diseases*. 100pp. 1981. Saffron Walden, Essex: Health Science Press. First published in 1967.
   Excellent. Twelve epidemic diseases and their treatment are surveyed.

428 Shepherd, D. *The magic of the minimum dose*. 214pp. 1979. Holsworthy, Devon: Health Science Press. First published in 1937.
   Very clearly written.

429 Shepherd, D. *More magic of the minimum dose: experiences and cases*. 286pp. 1980. Holsworthy, Devon: Health Science Press.

430 Shepherd, D. *A physician's posy*. 256pp. 1981. Saffron Walden, Essex: Health Science Press. First published in 1949.

431 Shinghal, J.N. *Quick bed-side prescriber with notes on clinical relationship of remedies and homoeopathy in surgery*. 760pp. 1983. New Delhi, India: B. Jain.
   Popular with students.

432 Simpson, James Y. *Homoeopathy: its tenets and tendencies, theoretical,*

theological and therapeutical. 292pp. 1853. Edinburgh: Sutherland and Knox.

433   Sivaraman, P. *Asthma cured with homoeopathic medicines.* 106pp. 1982. New Delhi, India: B. Jain.

434   Sivaraman, P. *A concise repertory of aggravations and ameliorations.* 320pp. 1980. New Delhi, India: B. Jain.

435   Sivaraman, P. *Corrections and additions to Kent's 'Repertory' (6th edition).* 456pp. 1982. New Delhi, India: World Homoeopathic Links.

436   Sivaraman, P. *Ear, nose and throat troubles cured with homoeopathic medicines.* 686pp. 1981. New Delhi, India: B. Jain.

437   Sivaraman, P. *Epilepsy cured with homoeopathic medicines.* 96pp. 1982. New Delhi, India: B. Jain.

438   Sivaraman, P. *Haemorrhoids cured by homoeopathic medicines.* 150pp. 1979. New Delhi, India: B. Jain.

439   Sivaraman, P. *Lady be healthy: female diseases with their homoeopathic medicines.* 397pp. 1980. New Delhi, India: B. Jain.
A materia medica and repertory. A useful work.

440   Skinner, Thomas. *Homoeopathy; specially in its relation to the diseases of women, or gynecology.* 104pp. 1903. London: W. H. Aukland.

441   Smith, Trevor. *An encyclopaedia of homoeopathy.* 280pp. 1983. Worthing, Sussex: Insight Publishing Co.

442   Smith, T. *Homoeopathic medicine.* 256pp. 1982. Wellingborough, Northamptonshire: Thorsons.
A detailed self-help guide.

443   Smith, T. *The homoeopathic treatment of emotional illness.* 208pp. 1983. Wellingborough, Northamptonshire: Thorsons.
Includes a self-help guide.

444   Smith, T. *Understanding homoeopathy: a simple and new approach to the fundamentals and basis of the method.* 98pp. 1983. Worthing, Sussex: Insight Publishing Co.

445   Smith, T. *A woman's guide to homoeopathic medicine.* 192pp. 1984. Wellingborough, Northamptonshire: Thorsons.

446 Snelling, Frederick G. (editor). *Hull's Jahr: a new manual of homoeopathic practice: repertory. With an appendix of the new remedies by C.J. Hempel.* 804pp. 1874. New York: Boericke and Tafel.

447 Snelling, F.G. (editor). *Hull's Jahr: a new manual of homoeopathic practice: symptomology. With an appendix of the new remedies by C.J. Hempel.* 1272pp. 1885. Philadelphia, Pennsylvania: Boericke and Tafel.

448 Speight, Leslie J. (compiler). *Homoeopathy and immunization.* 12pp. 1982. Saffron Walden, Essex: Health Science Press.
A practical booklet.

449 Speight, Phyllis. *Arnica the wonder herb.* 45pp. 1977. Holsworthy, Devon: Health Science Press.

450 Speight, P. *Before calling the doctor.* 47pp. 1976. London: C.W. Daniel.
A very concise handbook.

451 Speight, P. *A comparison of the chronic miasms: psora, pseudo-psora, syphilis, sycosis.* 52pp. 1977. London: C. W. Daniel.
An important work for the practitioner.

452 Speight, P. *Homoeopathic remedies for children.* 96pp. 1983. Saffron Walden, Essex: C.W. Daniel.
A clear, concise book.

453 Speight, P. *Homoeopathy: a practical guide to natural medicine.* 187pp. 1982. London: Granada.
A well written introduction.

454 Speight, P. *Overcoming rheumatism and arthritis.* 64pp. 1974. Wellingborough, Northamptonshire: Thorsons.
Includes herbs and naturopathy as well as homoeopathy.

455 Speight, P. *A study course in homoeopathy.* 1979. 145pp. Holsworthy, Devon: Health Science Press.

456 Stapf, Ernst (edited by and collected by) (translated by C.J. Hempel). *Additions to the materia medica pura.* 292pp. 1846. New York: William Radde.

457 Stearns, Guy Beckley and Edgar D. Evia. *The physical basis of*

homoeopathy and a new synthesis. 1982. New Delhi, India: World Homoeopathic Links.

458   Stephenson, James A. *A doctor's guide to helping yourself with homoeopathic remedies.* 197pp. 1983. Wellingborough, Northamptonshire: Thorsons.
Helpful introduction to homoeopathic self-care.

459   Stephenson, J.A. *Hahnemannian provings 1924–1959. A materia medica and repertory.* 155pp. 1963. Bombay, India: Roy and Company.
A comprehensive collection, and useful bibliography, based mainly on the *British Homeopathic Journal.*

460   Swan, Samuel. *A materia medica containing provings and clinical verifications of nosodes and morbific products.* 121pp. 1888. New York: Press of Pusey and Co.

461   Talcott, Selden Haines. *Mental diseases and their modern treatment.* 360pp. 1901. New York: Boericke and Runyon.
A series of lectures.

462   Teste, A. *The homoeopathic materia medica.* 634pp. 1983. New Delhi, India: B. Jain. First published in 1854 in France.

463   Thomas, Henry (collected and arranged by). *Additions to the homoeopathic materia medica.* 104pp. 1858. London: Thomas Sanderson.

464   Thomas, H. *Arnica, calendula, cantharis as external remedies in accidents, with an appendix on the use of camphor.* 103pp. 1981. New Delhi, India: B. Jain.

465   Tyler, M.L. *Hahnemann's conception of chronic disease as caused by parasitic micro-organisms.* 32pp. 1933. London: John Bale, Sons and Danielsson.

466   Tyler, M.L. *Homoeopathic drug pictures.* 885pp. 1980. Holsworthy, Devon: Health Science Press. First published in 1942 in London.
A standard textbook for students of homoeopathy.

467   Tyler, M.L. *Homoeopathy: introductory lectures.* 28pp. n.d. London: British Homoeopathic Association.
Lectures originally given to train medical missionaries.

468   Tyler, M.L. *Pointers to the common remedies*. (9 volumes bound into one). 337pp. 1983. New Delhi, India: B. Jain.
The most useful quick-reference book. A classic.

469   Tyler, M.L. and John Weir. *Some of the outstanding homoeopathic remedies for acute conditions, injuries, etc. with special indications for their use.* 44pp. 1982. London: British Homoeopathic Association. First published *c.* 1942.

470   Tyler, M.L. and J. Weir. *Uses of the repertory and 'repertorising'.* 43pp. n.d. New Delhi, India: B. Jain.

471   Vannier, Léon (translated by Mark Clements). *Homoeopathy: human medicine.* 231pp. n.d. Holsworthy, Devon: Health Science Press. First published *c.* 1930.
An interesting philosophical discussion of homoeopathy.

472   Verma, S.P. *Practical handbook of gynaecology*. 255pp. 1973. New Delhi, India: B. Jain.
Excellent.

473   Verma, S.P. *Practical handbook of surgery: with homoeopathic therapeutics.* 567pp. 1974. New Delhi, India: B. Jain.
A comprehensive analysis.

474   Vithoulkas, George. *Homoeopathy: medicine of the new man. A complete introduction to the revolutionary natural system of medicine whose time has come.* 154pp. 1983. New York: Arco.
This edition is highly recommended.

475   Vithoulkas, G. *The science of homoeopathy.* I: *The laws and principles of cure.* II: *The principles of homoeopathy in practical application.* 348pp. 1980. New York: Grove Press.
A very comprehensive and up-to-date book.

476   Voegeli, Adolph (translated by G.A. Dudley). *Homeopathic prescribing.* 94pp. 1976. Wellingborough, Northamptonshire: Thorsons.
An excellent home manual.

477   Voorhoeve, *Dr.* (translated, revised and edited by T. Miller Neatby). *Dr. Voorhoeve's homoeopathy in practice.* 448pp. n.d. London: The Homoeopathic Publishing Co.

478   Ward, James William. *The principles and scope of homoeopathy.* 73pp. 1925. Name of publisher not given.
Six lectures delivered during March and April 1925 at the University of California Training School for Nurses.

479   Ward, J.W. *Unabridged dictionary of the sensations 'as if'.* Volume 1: *Pathogenic.* Volume 2: *Clinical and bibliography.* 1801pp. 1983. New Delhi, India: B. Jain. First published in 1939 in one volume, in San Francisco.

480   Weiner, Michael and Kathleen Gross. *The complete book of homeopathy.* 310pp. 1982. London: Bantam Books.
A comprehensive introductory book for lay people.

481   Weir, John. *Hahnemann on homoeopathic philosophy.* 22pp. n.d. London: John Bale, Sons and Danielsson Ltd.
A reprint of a Compton Burnett Lecture published *c.* 1928.

482   Weir, J. *Homoeopathy: a system of therapeutics.* 12pp. n.d. New Delhi, India: Sandhu.

483   Weir, J. *The science and art of homoeopathy.* 14pp. 1927. London: British Homoeopathic Association.
A transcription of a talk.

484   Wells, P.P. *Essays on the treatment of diarrhoea and dysentery.* 211pp. n.d. Calcutta, India: Sett Dey.

485   Wells, P.P. and C.M.F. von Boenninghausen. *Intermittent fever.* 262pp. 1937. Calcutta, India: Sett Dey. Dr. Wells' *Intermittent fever* (first published in 1891 in Philadelphia) is bound together with the *Repertory* of von Boenninghausen.

486   Wheeler, Charles E. *The case for homoeopathy.* 98pp. 1933. London: British Homoeopathic Association.

487   Wheeler, C.E. and J.D. Kenyon. *An introduction to the principles and practice of homoeopathy.* 371pp. 1982. Saffron Walden, Essex: C.W. Daniel. First published in London in 1948.
An important work.

488   Whitmont, Edward C. *Psyche and substance: essays on homoeopathy in the light of Jungian psychology.* 190pp. 1980. Richmond, California: North Atlantic Books.

489   Williamson, Walter. *Diseases of females and children and their homoeopathic treatment.* 256pp. 1974. New Delhi, India: B. Jain.
A comprehensive work.

490   Woodbury, Benjamin C. *Homoeopathic materia medica for nurses.* 205pp. 1922. Chicago, Illinois: Ehrhart and Karl.

491   Woods, H. Fergie. *Essentials of homoeopathic prescribing.* 77pp. 1981. Holsworthy, Devon: Health Science Press.

492   Woods, H.F. *Homoeopathic treatment in the nursery.* 12pp. n.d. London: British Homoeopathic Association.
Includes some general information as well as specific sections on the ailments and their remedies.

493   Woodward, A.W. *Constitutional therapeutics.* 557pp. 1977. New Delhi, India: B. Jain. First published in 1903 in Philadelphia.

494   Worcester, Samuel. *Repertory to the modalities in their relations to temperature, air, water, winds, weather and seasons.* 168pp. 1983. New Delhi, India: World Homoeopathic Links. First published in 1880.

495   Yeldham, Stephen. *Homoeopathy in acute diseases.* 276pp. 1850. London: H. Baillière.

496   Yeldham, S. *Homoeopathy in venereal disease.* 192pp. n.d. New Delhi, India: World Homoeopathic Links. First published in 1880.
Interesting historically. Contains case studies.

497   Yingling, W.A. *Accoucheur's emergency manual.* 303pp. 1936. Calcutta, India: Sett Dey. First published in 1894.
Designed for practitioners.

Herbal Medicine

498 Allport, Noel S. *The chemistry and pharmacy of vegetable drugs.* 264pp. 1944. London: George Newnes.

499 Arber, Agnes. *Herbals: their origin and evolution. A chapter in the history of botany, 1470–1670.* 325pp. 1938. Cambridge: Cambridge University Press.

500 Back, Philippa. *Herbs about the house.* 94pp. 1977. London: Darton, Longman and Todd.
   Looks at all the uses of herbs: medicinal, cleansing, culinary, etc.

501 Banister, J. *The workes of the famous chyrurgian Mr. Iohn Banester, by him digested into five works.* 1633. London: Thomas Harper.

502 Barton, Benjamin Smith. *Collection for an essay towards a materia medica of the United States.* 83pp. 1810. (3rd edition). Philadelphia, Pennsylvania: published for E. Earle.

503 Bartram, Thomas. *Nature's plan for your health.* 245pp. 1975. Poole, Dorset: Blandford Press.

504 Beach, Wooster. *The British and American reformed practice of medicine embracing a treatise on the cause, systems and treatment of diseases generally.* 1071pp. 1859. Birmingham: Thomas Simmons.
   A standard work for present-day consulting herbalists.

505 Beach, W. *The family physician, or, the reformed system of medicine: on vegetable or botanical principles, being a compendium of 'the American practice of medicine'.* 782pp. 1844. New York: By author.

506   Beckett, Sarah. *Herbs for clearing the skin.* 64pp. 1983. Wellingborough, Northamptonshire: Thorsons.
Alphabetically organized according to herbs.

507   Beckett, S. *Herbs for feminine ailments.* 63pp. 1973. Wellingborough, Northamptonshire: Thorsons.
A practical guide.

508   Beckett, S. *Herbs for prostate and bladder troubles.* 63pp. 1979. Wellingborough, Northamptonshire: Thorsons.
An alphabetically arranged discussion of twenty-five herbs.

509   Beckett, S. *Herbs for rheumatism and arthritis.* 62pp. 1981. Wellingborough, Northamptonshire: Thorsons.
A practical guide.

510   Beckett, S. *Herbs to soothe your nerves.* 64pp. 1979. Wellingborough, Northamptonshire: Thorsons.
A useful, practical compendium.

511   Beedell, Suzanne. *Herbs for health and beauty.* 174pp. 1972. London: Sphere Books.

512   Benn, Thomas. *The botanic doctor's advisor.* 96pp. 1911. Leeds: Fred R. Spark and Son.

513   Bethel, May. *The healing power of herbs.* 160pp. 1974. North Hollywood, Calfornia: Wilshire Book Company.
An excellent book tracing uses and properties of various herbs.

514   Bianchini, Francesco and Corbetta Francesco. *Health plants of the world: atlas of medicinal plants.* 242pp. 1977. New York: Newsweek Books.
A beautiful book. Recommended.

515   Bigelow, Jacob. *American medicinal botany.* 3 volumes. 1817–20. Boston, Massachusetts: Name of publisher not given.
An account of the general history of American herbalism. An important work.

516   Binding, G.J. *About aromatic herbs.* 63pp. 1972. Wellingborough, Northamptonshire: Thorsons.

517   Binding, G.J. *About comfrey: the forgotten herb.* 63pp. 1981.
Wellingborough, Northamptonshire: Thorsons.
   A book of general interest.

518   Binding, G.J. *About garlic: the supreme herbal remedy.* 63pp. 1981.
Wellingborough, Northamptonshire: Thorsons.

519   Blate, Michael. *The G–Jo Institute manual of medicinal herbs.* 137pp.
1983. London: Routledge and Kegan Paul.
   Covers over seventy medicinal herbs.

520   Blythe, Peter. *Drugless medicine.* 176pp. 1974. London: Arthur
Barker.
   A study of alternative therapies including herbal medicine: there is
   a whole chapter on the Hoxsey cure for cancer, which uses herbs.

521   Bowker, W. *A brief treatise on various ailments and their treatment by
nature's remedies.* 48pp. 1890s. Bradford: The Medical Institute.

522   Bowness, Charles. *The Romany way to health.* 96pp. Wellingbor-
ough, Northamptonshire: Thorsons.
   Discusses the Romany usage of medicinal plants and gives the
   Romany cure for a number of common complaints.

523   Boxer, Arabella and Philippa Black. *The herb book.* 224pp. 1980.
London: Mayflower Books.
   Describes the history and traditions of herbs and explains their uses
   and cultivation.

524   British Herbal Medicine Association's Scientific Committee.
British Herbal Pharmacopoeia. Part 1: 242pp. 1976. Part 2: 248pp. 1976.
Part 3: 110pp. 1981. London: British Herbal Medicine Association.
   Recommended.

525   British Pharmaceutical Codex, The. 1791pp. 1934. London:
The Pharmaceutical Press.
   The best edition for instructions on the preparation of a large
   number of herbs now disappeared from codices.

526   Broadbent, John. *Botanic 'multum in parvo', being an index of
diseases and their treatment with botanic remedies.* 90pp. 1896. Melbourne,
Victoria: John Broadbent and Sons.

527   Brook, Richard. *A new family herbal: being a description of all the
plants which are useful to man.* 518pp. 1850s. London: W. M. Clark.

528   Brooker, S.G. and R.C. Cooper. *New Zealand medicinal plants. A handbook of the Auckland War Memorial Museum.* 46pp. 1962. Auckland, New Zealand: Unity Press Ltd.

529   Brown, O. Phelps. *The complete herbalist; or the people are their own physicians by the use of natural remedies.* 504pp. 1907. London: W. Foulsham. First published in 1893.
Of historical interest and a book that is still respected today.

530   Bruton, T. Lauder. *A textbook of pharmacology, therapeutics and materia medica.* 1261pp. 1893. London: Macmillan and Co. This 3rd edition has a supplement containing the additions, 1891, to the *British Pharmacopoeia*. The book was first published in 1885.

531   Buchan, William. *Domestic medicine or, a treatise on the prevention and cure of diseases by regimen and simple medicine.* 624pp. 1797. Edinburgh: Balfour, Auld and Smellie.
Of historical interest.

532   Buchan, W. *The new domestic medicine.* 511pp. 1830. London: W. Lewis.
A newer version of *Domestic medicine.*

533   Buchman, Dian Dincin. *Feed your face: a complete herbal guide to natural beauty and health.* 146pp. 1973. London: Gerald Duckworth and Co.

534   Buchman, D.D. *Herbal medicine: the natural way to get well and stay well.* 299pp. 1983. London: Rider and Company in association with The Herb Society.
Contains a great deal of practical information: how to make herbal medicine, collection and storage of herbs, suppliers of herbs, and so on.

535   Budge, Ernest Wallis. *The divine origin of the craft of the herbalist.* 96pp. 1928. London: The Society of Herbalists.
Traces the history of herbs back to antiquity.

536   Ceres. *The healing power of herbal teas: a guide to growing, preparing and using herbs for alleviating minor ailments.* 128pp. 1984. Wellingborough, Northamptonshire: Thorsons.

537   Ceres. *Herbal teas, tisanes, and lotions.* 128pp. 1981. Wellingborough, Northamptonshire: Thorsons.

Contains a guide to growing, preparing and using herbs for making stimulating tonics, soothing infusions and refreshing drinks.

538   Ceres. *Herbal teas for health and healing: self-treatment with nature's medicine*. 128pp. 1984. Wellingborough, Northamptonshire: Thorsons. Describes a wide range of tea-making herbs and explains their therapeutic properties.

539   Ceres. *Herbs and fruit for vitamins*. 65pp. 1975. Wellingborough, Northamptonshire: Thorsons.
   A good general-interest book.

540   Ceres. *Herbs for acidity and gastric ulcers*. 63pp. 1976. Wellingborough, Northamptonshire: Thorsons.
   Discusses twenty herbs in alphabetical order.

541   Ceres. *Herbs for first-aid and minor ailments*. 64pp. 1972. Boulder, Colorado: Shambhala Publications.
   A useful compendium, alphabetically arranged by the herbs.

542   Ceres. *Herbs for healthy hair*. 62pp. 1983. Wellingborough, Northamptonshire: Thorsons.
   Twenty herbs for hair care.

543   Ceres. *Herbs for indigestion*. 62pp. 1981. Wellingborough, Northamptonshire: Thorsons.

544   Ceres. *Herbs to help you sleep*. 62pp. 1981. Wellingborough, Northamptonshire: Thorsons.

545   Chemist and Druggist, The. *Pharmaceutical botany: botany without tears*. 300pp. 1920. London: The Chemist and Druggist.

546   Christopher, J. R. *Childhood diseases*. 205pp. 1976. Provo, Utah: Dr. John Christopher.
   Christopher, an esteemed herbalist in the United States, applies his herbal theories and formulas to childhood diseases.

547   Christopher, J.R. *School of natural healing*. 654pp. 1976. Provo, Utah: Dr. John Christopher.
   A comprehensive herbal work and encyclopaedia. Highly recommended for all who practise herbal medicine.

548   Clymer, Swinburne R. *The medicines of nature: the Thomsonian*

system. 205pp. 1960. Quakertown, Pennsylvania: The Humanitarian Society.

A classic reference work offering an excellent therapeutic basis for the application and use of herbal substances.

549   Coffin, Albert Isiah. *A botanic guide to health and the natural pathology of disease*. 374pp. 1848. Manchester: Wm. Irvin.

550   Coffin, A. I. *Medical botany: a course of lectures*. 223pp. 1850. London: W.B. Ford.

Covers the history of medicine herbs and their uses.

551   Colby, Benjamin. *Guide to health: the Thomsonian system of natural medicine*. 181pp. n.d. Orem, Utah: BiWorld. First published in 1846.

552   Colin, Jane. *Herbs and spices*. 176pp. 1980. London: Arlington Books.

A complete guide to all readily available herbs and spices.

553   Conrow, Robert and Arlene Hecksell. *Herbal pathfinders: voices of the herb renaissance*. 286pp. 1984. Santa Barbara, California: Woodbridge Press.

Interviews with leading herbalists.

554   Conway, David. *The magic of herbs*. 158pp. 1973. New York: E. P. Dutton.

Covers a very wide range of herbs.

555   Cook, William H. *Woman's herbal book of health: a textbook for the herbal practitioner and a guide for the wife, mother and nurse*. 1920. Southport: W.H. Webb.

556   Coon, Nelson. *The dictionary of useful plants*. 304pp. 1974. London: Rodale.

A compendium of information on hundreds of plants found in the United States. A clearly written account.

557   Coon, N. *Using plants for healing*. 284pp. 1979. Emmaus, Pennsylvania: Rodale.

A brief history and general introduction to herbal medicine, including a practical guide to uses and preparation of simple remedies.

558   Coon, N. *Using wild and wayside plants*. 284pp. 1980. New York: Dover Publications.

Describes many common wild plants and oraganizes them by type.

559   Crow, W. B. *The occult properties of herbs.* 64pp. 1969. New York: Samuel Weiser.
An overview.

560   Culpeper, Nicholas. *Culpeper's British herbal and complete English physician.* 2 volumes. 1805. London: H. Hogg.

561   Culpeper, N. (edited by David Potterton). *Culpeper's colour herbal.* 224pp. 1983. Slough: W. Foulsham.
Provides a link between the charm and elegance of seventeenth century scholarship and the resurgence of interest in herbal medicine. In this book Culpeper's conclusions 'have been evaluated against modern research and practice to produce an up-to-date English herbal'.

562   Culpeper, N. *Culpeper's complete herbal consisting of a comprehensive description of nearly all herbs with their medicinal properties and direction for compounding the medicines extracted from them.* 430pp. n.d. Slough: W. Foulsham.
A facsimile of the original herbal.

563   Culpeper, N. *Culpeper's everyman his own doctor.* 384pp. 1859. Halifax: Milner and Sowerby.

564   Culpeper, N. *Culpeper's herbal remedies.* 128pp. 1973. North Hollywood, California: Wilshire Book Company.
An adaptation of *Culpeper's complete herbal* intended for modern use.

565   Culpeper, N. *Culpeper's last legacy.* 2 parts. 1662. London: N. Brook.

566   Culpeper, N. (edited by C.F. Leyel). *The English physician and complete herbal.* 158pp. 1972. North Hollywood, California: Wilshire Book Company. This edition was first published in 1961 in London. Culpeper's book was first published in 1652 as *The English physician, or, an astrologo-physical discourse of the vulgar herbs of this nation. Being a compleat method of physick, whereby a man may preserve his body in health; or cure himself, being sick.*

567   Culpeper, N. *Pharmacopoeia Londinenis, or, the London dispensatory.* 377pp. 1659. London: Printed by Peter Cole.

568   Daisley, Gilda. *The illustrated book of herbs.* 128pp. 1982. London: Ebury Press.
Describes forty-one herbs.

569   Dale, W. *The principles and practice of the botanic system of medicine: a guide to the understanding of the nature of disease, its prevention and cure by the use of simple, safe and sanative means.* 176pp. 1855. Glasgow: Murray and Son.

570   Davies, Jill. *Herbal teas.* 144pp. To be published February 1985. London: Frederick Muller.

571   Davies, J. *The living herbalist: first steps towards natural healing.* To be published in March 1985. London: Hamish Hamilton.

572   Densmore, Frances. *How Indians use wild plants for food, medicine and crafts.* 397pp. 1974. New York: Dover Publications.

573   Dixon, Pamela. *Ginseng.* 101pp. 1976. London: Gerald Duckworth and Co.
A well researched book for the general reader.

574   Doole, Louise Evans. *Herbs for health: how to grow and use them.* 128pp. 1962. North Hollywood, California: Wilshire Book Company.

575   Duran-Reynals, M. L. *The fever bark tree: the pageant of quinine.* 251pp. 1914. London: W.H. Allen.
Of historical interest.

576   Eagle, Robert. *Herbs, useful plants.* 96pp. 1981. London: British Broadcasting Corporation.
Looks at the use of herbs through the centuries, including today.

577   Ellingwood, Finley and John Uri Lloyd. *Materia medica and therapeutics.* 1905. Chicago, Illinois: Medical Times.
Highly recommended.

578   Ellingwood, F. and J.U. Lloyd. *New American materia medica, therapeutics and pharmacognosy.* 1919. Evanstan, Illinois: Ellingwood Therapeutist.
A classic, and highly recommended.

579   Fernie, W.T. *Meals medicinal: with 'herbal simples' (of edible parts): curative foods from the cook: in place of drugs from the chemist.* 781pp. 1905. Bristol: John Wright.

580   Flück, Hans (translated by J. M. Rowson). *Medicinal plants and their uses.* 188pp. 1976. London: W. Foulsham.

A thoroughly practical guide to the most important medicinally used plants.

581 Foley, Daniel (editor). *Herbs for use and for delight*. 323pp. 1974. New York: Dover Publications.
A collection of articles by amateur scientists, selected from *The Herbalist* (the annual publication of The Herb Society of America).

582 Fox, William. *The working man's model family botanic guide or, every man his own doctor*. 304pp. 1904. Sheffield: William Fox and Sons.
The first popular book written on the subject.

583 Fulder, Stephen. *About ginseng: the magical herb of the East*. 64pp. 1981. Wellingborough, Northamptonshire: Thorsons.
An introductory discussion.

584 Fulder, S. *An end to ageing: traditional and modern ways of extending healthy life*. 112pp. 1983. Wellingborough, Northamptonshire: Thorsons.

585 Fulder, S. *The root of being: ginseng and the pharmacology of harmony*. 328pp. 1980. London: Hutchinson.
Traces the history of non-toxic medicines such as ginseng from early history.

586 Gabriel, Ingrid. *Herb identifier and handbook*. 256pp. 1975. New York: Sterling Publishing Company.
Over one hundred herbs are described.

587 Gerard, John. *The herbal or general history of plants: the complete 1633 edition as revised and enlarged by Thomas Johnson*. 1723pp. 1975. London: Constable.
Gerard's herbal, first published in 1597, has long been the most famous English herbal.

588 Gordon, Lesley. *Green magic: flowers, plants and herbs in lore and legend*. 200pp. 1977. London: Ebury Press.
A good, informative book.

589 Gosling, Nalda. *Herbs for bronchial troubles*. 64pp. 1981. Wellingborough, Northamptonshire: Thorsons.

590 Gosling, N. *Herbs for colds and flu*. 64pp. 1980. Wellingborough, Northamptonshire: Thorsons.

591 Gosling, N. *Herbs for constipation and other bowel disorders.* 64pp. 1982. Wellingborough, Northamptonshire: Thorsons.

592 Gosling, N. *Herbs for headaches and migraine.* 62pp. 1980. Wellingborough, Northamptonshire: Thorsons.

593 Gosling, N. *Herbs for the heart and circulation.* 62pp. 1980. Wellingborough, Northamptonshire: Thorsons.

594 Grieve, Maud. *A modern herbal* 912pp. 1982. Harmondsworth, Middlesex: Penguin.
Very thorough but enjoyable to read.

595 Griffith-Jones, Joy. *The virtuous weed.* 44pp. 1977. London: Blond and Briggs.
Descriptions with drawings of weeds and their uses, including medicinal.

596 Griggs, Barbara. *Green pharmacy: a history of herbal medicine.* 379pp. 1981. London: Jill Norman and Hobhouse.
Recommended. Informative and very enjoyable.

597 Griggs, B. *The home herbal: a handbook of simple remedies.* 160pp. 1983. London: Jill Norman and Hobhouse.

598 Grigson, Geoffrey Edward Harvey. *A herbal of all sorts.* 96pp. 1959. London: Phoenix House.

599 Hall, Dorothy, *The book of herbs.* 211pp. 1981. London: Pan Books.
A guide to herbs and their natural use in cooking, health and beauty.

600 Hall, D. *The herb tea book.* 109pp. 1981. New Canaan, Connecticut: Keats.
Describes many herbal teas and explains their healing and strengthening properties.

601 Hand, Wayland D. (editor). *American folk medicine.* 347pp. 1976. Berkeley, California: University of California Press.
Developing out of the proceedings of the UCLA Conference on American Folk Medicine, this is the first general collection of studies on folk medicine in North America.

602   Hanssen, Maurice. *About devil's claw: the natural and safe treatment of rheumatism and arthritis.* 64pp. 1979. Wellingborough, Northamptonshire: Thorsons.

603   Harding, A.R. *Ginseng and other medicinal plants.* 367pp. 1908. Mokelumne Hill, California: Health Research.
   The first discussion of ginseng and still one of the most comprehensive.

604   Harmer, Juliet. *The magic of herbs and flowers. An illustrated manuscript celebrating their healing properties.* Pages not numbered. 1980. London: Macmillan London.

605   Harper-Shove, F. *Prescriber and clinical repertory of medicinal herbs: an encyclopaedia of cures using herbs.* 228pp. 1982. Saffron Walden, Essex: C.W. Daniel.
   The first repertory to be published for herbalists.

606   Harriman, Sarah. *The book of ginseng.* 154pp. 1977. New York: Jove Publications.
   Looks at history and folk lore as well as reporting the latest research into its uses and information on buying, growing and using ginseng.

607   Harris, Ben Charles. *Better health with culinary herbs.* 163pp. 1971. Barre, Massachusetts: Barre Publishers.
   A detailed survey.

608   Harris, B.C. *The compleat herbal.* 243pp. 1980. New York: Larchmont Books.
   A comprehensive guide to medical plants.

609   Harris, B.C. *Ginseng: what it is, what it can do for you.* 126pp. 1978. New Canaan, Connecticut: Keats.
   A comprehensive look at ginseng.

610   Harris, B.C. *Kitchen medicines.* 80pp. 1955. Worcester, Massachusetts: By author.
   Alphabetically listed.

611   Harvey, Gideon. *The family physician and house apothecary.* 165pp. 1678. London: Printed for 'T.R.' No other details given. First published in 1676.

612 Harvey, Jack. *Herbs.* 96pp. 1978. London: Macdonald Educational.
A look at many aspects of herbs.

613 Hatfield, Audrey Wynne. *How to enjoy your weeds.* 116pp. 1972. London: Fredrick Muller.
Alphabetically arranged selection of weeds including description, folklore and health uses.

614 Heffern, Richard. *The complete book of ginseng.* 127pp. 1976. Millbrae, California: Celestial Arts.
A comprehensive presentation.

615 Heffern, R. *The herb buyer's guide.* 187pp. 1973. New York: Pyramid Publications.
The only available guide to the purchase, processing and use of herbs.

616 Heffern, R. *Secrets of the mind-altering plants of Mexico.* 204pp. 1974. New York: Pyramid Publications.
A detailed study.

617 Henslow, G. *The uses of British plants traced from antiquity to the present day.* 190pp. 1905. London: Lovell, Reeve and Co.

618 Hessayon, D.G. *Be your own garden doctor.* 34pp. 1978. Waltham Cross, Hertfordshire: Pan Britannica Industries.

619 Hessayon, D.G. *Be your own vegetable doctor.* 34pp. 1978. Waltham Cross, Hertfordshire: Pan Britannica Industries.

620 Hewlett-Parsons, J. *Herbs, health and healing.* 94pp. 1981. Wellingborough, Northamptonshire: Thorsons.
Recommended as a good overview.

621 Hill, *Sir* John. *The family herbal: or an account of all those English plants, which are remarkable for their virtues and of the drugs which are produced by vegetables of other countries; with their description and their uses, as proved by experience.* 440pp. 1789. Bungay: Brightly and Kinnersley.
Beautifully illustrated.

622 Hills, Lawrence D. *Comfrey: past present and future.* 253pp. 1976. London: Faber and Faber.
History, research, medicinal use.

623   Hoffmann, David. *The holistic herbal: a herbal celebrating the wholeness of life.* 271pp. 1983. Findhorn, Scotland: Findhorn Press.
Shows how herbs can be applied to patterns of disease and specific conditions.

624   Hool, Richard Lawrence. *British wild herbs and common plants, their uses in medicine: a guide to the most common and most useful non-poisonous British wild herbs and their medicinal virtues and applications to various complaints.* 180pp. 1924. Southport: W. H. Webb. Abridged from *The standard guide to non-poisonous herbal medicine* (edited by W.H. Webb).

625   Hou, Joseph. *The myth and the truth about ginseng.* 245pp. 1978. London: Thomas Yoseloff.
An extensive discussion.

626   Huibers, Jaap. *Herbs for kidneys, skin and eyes.* 64pp. 1981. Wellingborough, Northamptonshire: Thorsons.

627   Huson, Paul. *Mastering herbalism.* 371pp. 1974. New York: Stein and Day.
A well-written, unusual account.

628   Hutchens, Alma R. *Indian herbology of North America.* 382pp. 1974. Ontario, Canada: MERCO.
The definitive work on the subject, highly recommended for the serious student. Hutchens has done for Canadian herbalism what Potter did for British herbalism.

629   Hyatt, Richard. *Chinese herbal medicine: ancient art and modern science.* 160pp. 1978. London: Wildwood House.
A substantial exposition of Chinese herbal medicine as well as a detailed presentation of the many plants and drugs that comprise the Chinese pharmacopoeia.

630   Hylton, William and Josie A. Holton (editors). *The complete guide to herbs: how to grow and use nature's miracle plants.* 607pp. 1979. Aylesbury, Buckinghamshire: Rodale.
A herbal encyclopaedia.

631   Johnson, C. Pierpoint. *The useful plants of Great Britain: a treatise upon the native vegetables capable of application as food, medicine or in the arts and manufactures.* 350pp. n.d. London: Robert Hardwicke.
Of historical interest. Written in the 1860s.

632   Kadans, Joseph. *Encyclopedia of medicinal herbs*. 256pp. 1983. Wellingborough, Northamptonshire: Thorsons.
Very clearly presented.

633   Kelly, Howard A. *Some American medical botanists: commemorated in our botanical nomenclature*. 215pp. 1929. London: D. Appleton and Co.

634   Kerr, Ralph. *Herbalism through the ages*. 225pp. 1969. San Jose, California: AMORC.
Legends and folklore from antiquity to contemporary times.

635   Kirchner, H.E. *Nature's healing grasses*. 128pp. 1970. Riverside, California: H.C. White.
Vegetables, greens, herbs, described as medicines.

636   Kloss, Jethro. *Back to Eden*. 688pp. 1984. Santa Barbara: California: Woodbridge Press.
The most popular herbal.

637   Kourennoff, Paul M. (translated and edited by George St George). *Russian folk medicine*. 213pp. 1970. London: Pan Books.
Covers about 350 remedies.

638   Kreig, Margaret B. *Green medicine: the search for plants that heal*. 461pp. 1965. London: George G. Harrap.
Deals with the modern worldwide resurgence of scientific interest in medicinal plants.

639   Krochmal, Arthur and Connie Krochmal. *A guide to the medicinal plants of the United States*. 259pp. 1973. New York: Quadrangle.
A well organized account.

640   Langham, William. *The garden of health. Conteyning the ... virtues and properties of all kinds of simples and plants*. Pages not numbered. 1633. London: Thomas Harper. First published in 1578.

641   Law, Donald. *The concise herbal encyclopedia*. 266pp. 1973. Edinburgh: John Bartholomew and Son.
A comprehensive introduction to herbal medicine. Recommended.

642   Law, D. *Herbs for cooking and healing*. 104pp. 1970. London: W. Foulsham.

643   Law, D. *Herbs growing for health*. 223pp. 1972. New York: Arco.
Describes how to grow, use and recognize over 150 herbs.

644   La Wall, Charles H. *Four thousand years of pharmacy: an outline history*. 665pp. 1927. Philadelphia, Pennsylvania: J.B. Lippincott.

645   Lehane, Brendan. *The power of plants*. 288pp. 1977. London: John Murray.
Includes information on healing powers and also a modern herbal.

646   Levy, Juliette de Bairacli. *Common herbs for natural health*. 200pp. 1974. New York: Schocken Books.
An excellent herbal.

647   Levy, J. de B. *Herbal handbook for everyone*. 178pp. 1966. London: Faber and Faber.
For general use and for the beginner in herbal medicine.

648   Levy, J. de B. *The illustrated herbal handbook*. 224pp. 1982. London: Faber and Faber.
A well established book covering all aspects of herbs.

649   Lewis, Walter, P.F. Memory and Elvin Lewis. *Medicinal botany: plants affecting man's health*. 1977. New York: Wiley Interscience.
A clinically orientated volume of special interest to the physician and professional practitioner who want to learn more about the use of botanicals in medicine. Highly recommended.

650   Leyel, C.F. *Cinquefoil: herbs to quicken the five senses*. 268pp. 1957. London: Faber and Faber.

651   Leyel, C.F. *Compassionate herbs*. 224pp. 1946. London: Faber and Faber.
Herbs for wounds: antiseptics, astringents, pain controllers and herbs that allay fever.

652   Leyel, C.F. *Elixirs of life*. 221pp. 1948. London: Faber and Faber.
Covers herbs that prolong life.

653   Leyel, C.F. *Green medicine*. 324pp. 1930. London: Faber and Faber.
Herbs for different organs and parts of the body and the importance of chlorophyll in maintaining health.

654   Leyel, C.F. *Heart-ease: herbs for the heart, the ductless glands and the nerves*. 333pp. 1949. London: Faber and Faber.

655   Leyel, C.F. *The truth about herbs*. 106pp. 1954. London: Culpeper Press.
Addressing herself to the general reader, the author describes the history of herbalism and also her own work in medical herbalism.

656   Lingard, W. Burns and Alfred Hall. *Herbal prescriptions from a consultant's case book. And volatile oils.* 72pp. 1958. The National Institute of Medical Herbalists. No address given.

657   Lloyd, John Uri. *Origins and history of all the pharmacopoeial vegetable drugs, chemicals and preparations.* Volume 1: *Vegetables and drugs.* 449pp. 1921. Cincinnati, Ohio: The American Drug Manufacture Association.

658   Loewenfeld, C. and Philippa Back. *The complete book of herbs and spices.* 315pp. 1976. London: Pan Books.
Recommended to those who want a good, general introductory survey.

659   Loewenfeld, C. and P. Back. *Herbs for health and cookery.* 336pp. 1971. London: Pan Books.

660   Lucas, Richard. *Common and uncommon uses of herbs for healthful living.* 238pp. 1983. New York: Arco.
A comprehensive book for the beginner in this field.

661   Lucas, R. *Magic herbs for arthritis, rheumatism, and related ailments.* 248pp. 1981. Englewood Cliffs, New Jersey: Prentice-Hall.

662   Lucas, R. *The magic of herbs in daily living.* 263pp. 1979. West Nyack, New York: Parker Publishing Company.
Describes the uses of herbs in various conditions. Also includes information on the legendary occult powers of herbs.

663   Lucas, R. *Nature's medicines: the folklore, romance and value of herbal remedies.* 224pp. 1979. West Nyack, New York: Parker Publishing Company.
A fascinating account. Includes a report on what scientific research has shown about these old remedies.

664   Lucas, R. *Secrets of the Chinese herbalists.* 244pp. 1979. New York: Cornerstone Library (Simon and Schuster).
An excellent book on Chinese medicine.

665   Lust, Benedict. *About herbs: medicines from the meadows.* 64pp. 1980. Wellingborough, Northamptonshire: Thorsons.
A survey of the medicinal properties and folklore of the best-known herbs.

666   Lust, John. *The herb book.* 659pp. 1983. New York: Bantam Books.
This is one of the best contemporary herbals. A good book for the general reader.

667   Lyle, T.J. *Physio-medical therapeutics, materia medica and pharmacy.* 446pp. 1932. London: National Association of Medical Herbalists. First published in 1897.
Was originally one of the textbooks of the National Association of Medical Herbalists.

668   Mackinney, Loren. *Early medieval medicine: with special reference to France and Chartres.* 247pp. 1937. Baltimore: Publications of the Institute of the History of Medicine, Johns Hopkins University.

669   McLeod, Margot. *Handbook of herbs: growing, cooking, health etc.* 126pp. 1983. Kingswood, Surrey: Elliot Right Way Books.

670   Maisch, John M. *A manual of organic materia medica.* 556pp. 1892. London: Henry Kimpton.
Still of value to the serious student of herbal pharmacy.

671   Mansfield, William. *Histology of medicinal plants.* 305pp. 1916. London: Chapman and Hall.

672   Mausert, Otto. *Herbs.* 1974. Eugene, Oregon: Elaine M. Muhr.
An easy-to-read introduction to the use of herbal substances for healing.

673   Maxwell, Nicole. *Witch-doctor's apprentice.* 353pp. 1962. London: Victor Gollancz.

674   Mességué, Maurice. *Health secrets of herbs and plants.* 335pp. 1981. London: Pan Books.
A detailed and interesting encyclopaedia of herbal lore.

675   Mességué, M. *Of men and plants.* 298pp. 1972. London: Weidenfeld and Nicholson.
An autobiography.

676   Mességué, M. *Way to natural health and beauty.* 254pp. 1974. New York: Macmillan.
Contains good practical advice.

677   Meyer, Clarence. *American folk medicine.* 296pp. 1973. Bergenfield, New Jersey: New American Library.
A collection of early American remedies utilizing ingredients usually found at hand.

678   Meyer, Joseph E. *The herbalist.* 304pp. 1960. Hammond, Indiana: Hammond Book Co. First published in 1918.
One of the best-regarded older herbals.

679   Mez-Mangold, Lydia. *A history of drugs.* 1971. Basle, Switzerland: F. Hoffman-La Roche.

680   Miller, Amy Bess. *Shaker herbs.* 272pp. 1976. New York: Clarkson N. Potter.
The Shaker communities of eighteenth- and nineteenth-century America relied on herbal medicine and grew many of the herbs supplied to hospitals and pharmaceutical companies. This is a beautifully illustrated account of their involvement with herbs, together with a compendium of the herbs they sold with their own therapeutic notes and charming drawings.

681   Millspaugh, Charles. *American medicinal plants.* 828pp. 1974. New York: Dover Publications.
An unabridged reproduction of the 1892 edition, considered to be the definitive herbal of its day.

682   Mitton, F. and V. Mitton. *Mitton's practical modern herbal.* 134pp. 1982. London: W. Foulsham.
Deals with the history of herbal science and preparation and application of herbs, and has an A–Z guide to the most important herbs known to man.

683   Mitton, Mervyn. *Herbal remedies.* 64pp. 1984. Slough: W. Foulsham.
Offers simple, safe and effective remedies.

684   Morton, Julia F. *Major medicinal plants.* 1977. Springfield, Illinois: Charles C. Thomas.
An extremely well researched volume for the serious student of medicinal plants.

685   National Academy of Sciences. *Herbal pharmacology in the People's Republic of China.* 269pp. 1975. Washington, D.C.: National Academy of Sciences Printing and Publishing Office.
A highly technical volume.

686   Nebelkopf, Ethan. *The herbal connection: herbs, drug abuse and holistic health.* 188pp. 1981. Orem, Utah: BiWorld.

687   Neil, James F. *The New Zealand family herb doctor: a book on the botanic electic system of medicine, containing the latest discoveries in medicine and surgery, for the cure of disease; also, a description of the herbs, roots, arks, seeds, extracts, essential oils, etc.* 523pp. 1891. Dunedin: Mills Dick and Co., Lithographers.

688   Northcote, Lady Rosalind. *The book of herbs.* 212pp. 1912. London: The Bodley Head.
Medicinal uses are included.

689   Page, Robin. *Cures and remedies the country way.* 64pp. 1978. London: Davis-Poynter.

690   Pagel, Walter. *Paracelsus: an introduction to philosophical medicine in the era of the Renaissance.* 368pp. 1958. New York and Basle: S. Karger.

691   Pahlow, Mannfried. *Living medicine: the healing properties of plants.* 96pp. 1982. Wellingborough, Northamptonshire: Thorsons.
A clear, well organized guide to those plants that have been scientifically proven to have healing properties.

692   Palaiseul, Jean (translated by Pamela Swinglehurst). *Grandmother's secrets: her guide to health from plants.* 292pp. 1973. London: Barrie and Jenkins.

693   Palaiseul, J. (translated by P. Swinglehurst). *The green guide to health from plants.* 292pp. 1977. London: Book Club Associates.

694   Parkinson, John. *The theatre of plants, or an herball of a large extent.* 1755pp. 1640. London: Name of publisher not given.
Parkinson was the King's herbalist.

695   Parsons, J. Hewlett. *Herbs, health and healing.* 96pp. 1968. London: Thorsons.

696   Parvati, Jeannine. *Hygieia: a woman's herbal.* 248pp. 1979. London: Wildwood House.

The first book of its kind to interweave the ancient practice of herbalism with the women's consciousness movement and holistic health.

697   Pechey, John. *The English herbal of physical plants*. 96pp. 1951. London: Medical Publications.
An abridged reproduction of *The compleat herbal of physical plants*, 1694. Originally designed for general use, now of historical interest.

698   Peplow, Elizabeth. *The herb book: an A–Z of useful herbs*. 176pp. 1982. London: W. H. Allen.

699   Pereira, Jonathan (edited by R. Bentley and T. Rewood). *The elements of materia medica and therapeutics*. 2 parts. 1874. London: Name of publisher not given.

700   Petulengro, Gypsy (Xanier). *Romany remedies and recipes*. 75pp. 1935. London: Methuen.

701   Petulengro, Leon. *The roots of health: Romany lore for health and beauty*. 144pp. 1978. London: Pan Books.

702   Powell, Eric F. W. *About dandelions: the golden wonder herb*. 64pp. 1977. Wellingborough, Northamptonshire: Thorsons.
Designed for the lay person.

703   Powell, E.F.W. *Building a healthy heart: the magic of a wild berry*. 60pp. 1964. Rustington, Sussex: Health Science Press.

704   Powell, E.F.W. *Health secrets of all ages*. 131pp. n.d. Bognor Regis, Sussex: Health Science Press.
A wonderful book on health hygiene and well-tried herbal prescriptions for common troubles.

705   Powell, E.F.W. *Kelp: the health giver*. 40pp. 1970. Rustington, Sussex: Health Science Press.

706   Powell, E.F.W. *The modern botanic prescriber*. 136pp. 1965. London: L.N. Fowler.
Intended mainly for the intelligent housewife.

707   Priest, A.W. and L.R. Priest. *Herbal medication: a clinical and dispensary handbook*. 174pp. 1982. London: L.N. Fowler.

Meant for clinical students and newly qualified practitioners. Recommended.

708   Quelch, Mary Thorne. *Herbs for daily use.* 328pp. 1959. London: Faber and Faber.

709   Ranson, Florence. *British herbs.* 206pp. 1949. Harmondsworth, Middlesex: Penguin.
A manual of herb recognition written for the layman. Includes medicinal uses. A collector's item.

710   Rau, Henrietta A. Diers. *Healing with herbs: nature's way to better health.* 235pp. 1982. New York: Arco.
An encyclopaedic guide to the healing properties of a large number of herbs, primarily American. Recommended.

711   Roberts, Frank. *Herbal cures of duodenal ulcer and gall stones.* 45pp. 1981. Wellingborough, Northamptonshire: Thorsons. First published in 1969.

712   Roberts, F. *Modern herbalism for digestive disorders.* 160pp. 1981. Wellingborough, Northamptonshire: Thorsons. Originally published in 1957 as *The encyclopedia of digestive disorders.*
A very comprehensive guide to causes, symptoms, signs and herbal prescriptions, based on clinical experience.

713   Robinson, M. *Robinson's new family herbal and botanic physician.* 480pp. 1863. Halifax: William Nicholson and Sons.
Comprises a description of the medical properties and the mode of using British and foreign herbs. Of historical interest.

714   Rodale, J.I. *The hawthorn berry for the heart.* 125pp. 1971. Emmaus, Pennsylvania: Rodale.
An account of some of the medical accounts of the use of hawthorn in heart disease that have appeared this century.

715   Rohde, Eleanor Sinclair. *The old English herbals.* 243pp. 1971. New York: Dover Publications.
Originally published in 1922, discusses the important herbals from the eighth-century Anglo-Saxon ones up to modern times. Thoroughly recommended.

716   Rose, Jeanne. *Herbs and things.* 321pp. 1979. New York: Grosset and Dunlap.

An A–Z of diseases and the appropriate herbal cure based on the premise that plants are ruled by the planets.

717   Rowsell, Henry and Helen MacFarlane. *Modern bee herbal.* 128pp. 1978. Wellingborough, Northamptonshire: Thorsons.

718   Rubin, Stanley. *Medieval English medicine.* 232pp. 1974. Newton Abbot, Devon: David and Charles.

719   Ruddock, E.H. *Vitalogy: an encyclopaedia of health and home.* 110pp. 1931. Chicago, Illinois: Vitalogy Association.
In its time a standard textbook for American herbalists.

720   Rusholm, Peter (collated and edited by). *Country medicines.* 64pp. 1971. Rustington, Sussex: Health Science Press.
A simple alphabetical guide to the treatment of many common ailments by means of herbal and homoeopathic medicines that have been used successfully by the author.

721   Rutherford, Meg. *A pattern of herbs: herbs for goodness, food and health and how to identify and grow them.* 150pp. 1975. London: George Allen and Unwin.
Describes about forty-three herbs.

722   Said, Hakim Mohammed (editor). *Hamdard medicus.* 264pp. 1979. Hamdard, Pakistan: Hamdard Academy Foundation.
A collection of papers presented at a seminar held in Pakistan in 1979 on 'Pharmacy and Medicine through the Ages'.

723   Salmon, William. *The English herbal: or history of plants.* 1310pp. 1710. London: Name of publisher not given.
Of antiquarian interest but little practical application.

724   Sanecki, Kay N. *The complete book of herbs.* 247pp. 1975. London: Macdonald and Jane's.

725   Sanecki, K.N. *Discovering herbs.* 64pp 1982. Aylesbury, Buckinghamshire: Shire Publications.

726   Schauenberg, Paul and Ferdinand Paris. *Guide to medicinal plants.* 389pp. 1977. London: Lutterworth Press.
An introduction to the study of 401 medicinal plants.

727   Shepherd, Dorothy. *A physician's posy.* 256pp. 1981. Holsworthy, Devon: Health Science Press.

A compelling, sensitive account of healing the sick with herbal and homoeopathic preparations.

728   Shook, Edward E. *Advanced treatise on herbology*. 364pp. 1974. Mokelumne Hill, California: Health Research.
A fascinating and invaluable work.

729   Shook, E.E. *Elementary treatise in herbology*. 160pp. 1974. Beaumont, California: Trinity Center Press.
A series of lessons, which together form a basic course in herbology.

730   Silverrman, Maida. *A city herbal: a guide to the lore, legend, and usefulness of 34 plants that grow wild in the city*. 192pp. 1977. Westminster, Maryland: Random House.

731   Simons, Paul. *Garlic: the powerful panacea*. 96pp. 1982. Wellingborough, Northamptonshire: Thorsons.
Includes clinical evidence for garlic's medicinal properties, and details of its historical folklore.

732   Skelton, J. *The science and practice of medicine*. 768pp. 1904. London: National Association of Medical Herbalists.

733   Smith, Keith Vincent. *The illustrated earth garden herbal: a herbal companion*. 170pp. 1979. London: Elm Tree Books.

734   Smith, William. *Herbs for constipation*. 64pp. 1976. Wellingborough, Northamptonshire: Thorsons.
General advice and descriptions of a series of herbs and their usage.

735   Smith, W. *Herbs to ease bronchitis*. 63pp. 1973. Wellingborough, Northamptonshire: Thorsons.

736   Smith, W. *Wonders in weeds*. 187pp. 1977. Holsworthy, Devon: Health Science Press.
A practical A–Z of herbs, their uses and preparation.

737   Smythe, Benjamin Roth. *Killing cancer: the Jason Winters story*. 182pp. 1983. Boulder City, Nevada: Vinton Publishing.
The story of Winters' search for a herbal remedy for terminal cancer.

738   Speight, Phyllis. *Overcoming rheumatism and arthritis*. 64pp. 1974. Wellingborough, Northamptonshire: Thorsons.
Includes herbs as well as homoeopathy and naturopathy.

739   Spoerke, David G. *Herbal medications: a practical, descriptive guide book to the active principles of more than 200 medicinal herbs.* 192pp. 1980. Santa Barbara, California: Woodbridge Press.

740   Squire, Peter Wyatt. *Squire's companion to the latest edition of the 'British Pharmacopoeia'.* 1707pp. 1916. (19th edition). London: J. and A. Churchill.
    This work is not exclusive to herbs, but contains instructions for the preparation of standard extracts.

741   Stary, Frantisek and Jirasek, Vaclav. *Herbs.* 239pp. 1976. London: Hamlyn Paperbacks.
    A useful introduction to herbal medicine.

742   Step, Edward. *Herbs of healing: a book of British simples.* 116pp. 1950. London: Hutchinson. First published in 1926.

743   Strange, Richard le. *A history of herbal plants.* 325pp. 1977. London: Angus and Robertson.
    Surveys about 750 plants.

744   Stuart, Malcolm. *The encyclopaedia of herbs and herbalism.* 304pp. 1979. London: Orbis Publishing.
    Details of 420 of the most important herbs.

745   Stuart, M. (editor). *The colour dictionary of herbs and herbalism.* 160pp. 1982. London: Orbis Publishing.
    Describes 420 herbs, alphabetically arranged.

746   Swain, Tony (editor). *Plants in the development of modern medicine.* 1972. Cambridge, Massachusetts: Harvard University Press.

747   Swann, Claire. *Nettles. Healers of the wild.* 64pp. 1980. Wellingborough, Northamptonshire: Thorsons.
    Describes the nettle's remedial and nutritional properties.

748   Szekely, Edmund Bordeaux. *The book of herbs.* 46pp. 1975. San Diego, California: Academy Books.
    A brief compendium of diseases and remedies as well as a herbal materia medica.

749   Szekely, E.B. *Natural herb therapeutics.* 68pp. 1943. Tecate, California: Essene School of Life.
    Looks at many diseases and their herbal remedies.

750   Talbot, C.H. *Medicine in medieval England.* 222pp. 1967. London: Oldbourne.

751   Taylor, Gordon. *A handful of herbs.* Pages not numbered. 1976. London: Blond and Briggs.

752   Taylor, Norman. *Plant drugs that changed the world.* 275pp. 1966. London: George Allen and Unwin.
An account of the discovery and use of plants in medicine from earliest times to the present day.

753   Thesen, Karen. *Country remedies from pantry, field and garden.* 160pp. 1979. London: Pierrot.

754   Thomson, Robert. *Natural medicine.* 345pp. 1978. Highstown, New Jersey: McGraw-Hill.
An extremely comprehensive and lucid herbal.

755   Thomson, William A.R. *Healing plants: a modern herbal.* 208pp. 1980. London: Macmillan.
A handbook and dictionary of plants and their use in treating disease.

756   Thomson, W. A. R. *Herbs that heal.* 184pp. 1976. London: Adam and Charles Black.
Contends that herbs deserve serious attention from medics.

757   Thomson, W.A.R. *Medicines for the earth: a guide to healing plants.* 208pp. 1978. Highstown, New Jersey: McGraw-Hill.
An in-depth analysis of 247 medicinal herbs and flowers that grow in the wild.

758   Thomson, W.A.R. and Elizabeth Smith. *Healing herbs.* 64pp. 1978. London: British Broadcasting Corporation.
Compiled from listeners' responses to a 'You and yours' programme.

759   Thornton, Robert John. *A new family herbal: or popular account of the natures and properties of the various plants used in medicine, diet and the arts.* 917pp. 1810. London: Richard Phillips.

760   Tierra, Michael. *The way of herbs.* 240pp. 1980. San Francisco, California: Unity Press.

A simple, concise, clear guide to the healing properties and uses of herbs. Highly recommended.

761   Tobe, John H. *Proven herbal remedies*. 320pp. 1969. St. Catherines, Ontario: Provoker Press.
A very complete listing.

762   Tudor, Alice M. *A little book of healing herbs gathered from an old herball*. 74pp. 1927. London and Boston, Massachusetts: The Medici Society.
A lovely book.

763   Turner, William. *A new herball*. 2 parts. 1551. London: By author.

764   Twitchell, Paul. *Herbs: the magic healers*. 189pp. 1971. Menlo Park, California: Illuminated Way.
A very complete compendium.

765   *United States Dispensatory*. from 1,500 to 2,377pp. 1880s–1960. (5th–25th editions). Philadelphia: J. B. Lippincott.
The 25th edition was the last to include a section on herbs.

766   Usher, George. *A dictionary of plants used by man*. 1974. London: Constable.

767   Veissid, Jacques (translated by Nadia Legrand). *Folk medicine*. 226pp. 1979. London: Quartet Books.

768   Veninga, L. and Ben Zaricor. *Goldenseal/etc*. 193pp. 1976. Santa Cruz, California: Ruka Publications.
A very complete book.

769   Venzmer, Gerhard (translated by Marion Koenig) *Five thousand years of medicine*. 369pp. 1972. London: MacDonald and Co.

770   Vogel, A.C.A. *Nature doctor*. 392pp. 1977. Teufen, Switzerland: Verlag A. Vogel.
Contains many herbal remedies.

771   Vogel, Virgil J. *American Indian medicine*. 583pp. 1982. Norman, Oklahoma: University of Oklahoma Press.
Well written and informative. Its purpose is to show the effect of Indian practices on the white civilization.

772   Wagner, H. and D. Wolff (editors). *New natural products and plant drugs with pharmacological, biological or therapeutic activity.* 1977. Berlin, Heidelberg, New York. Proceedings of the First International Congress on Medicinal Plant Research.

773   Waller, John Augustine. *The new British domestic herbal.* 408pp. 1822. London: E. Cox and Son Printers.

774   Wallis, Thomas E. *A textbook of pharmacognosy.* 578pp. 1955. London: J. and A. Churchill.

775   Wallis, T.E. *Practical pharmacognosy.* 238pp. 1953. London: J. and A. Churchill.

776   Walters, W.D. *Wonderful herbal remedies.* 202pp. 1973. Swansea: Celtic Educational.
      Written by a pharmacist.

777   Ward, Harold. *Herbal manual. The medicinal, toilet, culinary and other uses of 130 of the most commonly used herbs.* 132pp. 1936. London: C.W. Daniel. Reissued in 1962 by L.N. Fowler (London).

778   Webb, Sarah A. *Diseases of women and children.* 176pp. n.d. Worcester: The National Association of Medical Herbalists of Great Britain.
      A period piece!

779   Webb, William Henry (editor). *Standard guide to non poisonous herbal medicine: an exposition of the British and American practice of reformed medicine, as inaugurated by Samuel Thomson in America, a century ago, and which broke down medical monopoly in that country. Also an account of the legal position of herbalism in England.* 371pp. 1916. Southport: W.H. Webb.

780   Weiner, Michael A. *Earth medicine, earth foods: plant remedies, drugs, and natural foods of the North American Indians.* 230pp. 1980. New York: Macmillan.

781   Weiner, M.A. *Weiner's herbal: the guide to herb medicine.* 224pp. 1980. New York: Stein and Day.
      Provides a readable layman's guide. Recommended.

782   Wesley, John (edited by William Paynter). *Primitive physic: or an easy and natural method of curing most diseases.* 80pp. 1958. Plymouth, Devon: Parade Printing Works.

A selection from the 1755 edition with additional cures and remedies from earlier editions.

783   Wesley, John. *Primitive remedies.* 142pp. 1984. Santa Barbara, California: Woodbridge Press.
The most popular work of John Wesley, the great Methodist reformer.

784   Wickham, Cynthia. *Common plants as natural remedies.* 144pp. 1981. London: Frederick Muller.
Simple remedies for minor ailments.

785   Withering, William. *An account of the foxglove.* 1785. London: Broomsleigh Press.

786   Woodville, William. *Medical botany.* 4 volumes. 824pp. 1810. London: William Phillips.

787   Woodward, Marcus. *The Gerard's herball. The essence thereof distilled by Marcus Woodward from the edition of T.H. Johnson 1636.* 303pp. 1927. London: Gerald Howe.

788   Woodward, M. (arranged by). *Leaves from Gerard's herball.* 305pp. 1972. London: Thorsons. Facsimile edition of the original 1927 volume, rearranged according to a garden calendar.

789   Wren, R.W. *Potter's handy prescriber: book of common ailments and appropriate treatments.* 64pp. n.d. London: Potter and Clarke. The first edition of this was for private circulation only.

790   Wren, R.W. (re-edited by). *Potter's new cyclopaedia of botanical drugs and preparations.* 416pp. 1975. London: C.W. Daniel. First published in 1907, edited by R.C. Wren.
A valuable reference book. Recommended.

791   Yemm, J.R. (editor). *The medical herbalist.* 125pp. 1977. North Hollywood, California: Wilshire Book Company.
A compilation of papers that appeared in the Journal of the National Institute of Medical Herbalists (then the Association) in the 1930s and 1940s. A fascinating collection.

Naturopathy

792 Abehsera, Michael. *The healing clay: amazing cures from the earth itself.* 126pp. 1977. Brooklyn, New York: Swan House.

793 Abrahams, Margery and Elsie M. Widdowson. *Modern dietary treatment.* 355pp. 1951. London: Baillière, Tindall and Cox. First published in 1937.

794 Abrahamson, E.M. and A.W. Pezet. *Body, mind and sugar.* 206pp. 1977. New York: Avon Books.
The first book to alert the public to the problem of low blood sugar.

795 Abramowski, O.L.M. *Fruitarian healing system.* 187pp. 1976. Durban, South Africa: Essence of Health.
The most complete discussion available.

796 Abravanel, Eliott D. and Elizabeth A. King. *Dr. Abravanel's body type diet and lifetime nutrition plan.* 256pp. 1983. New York: Bantam Books.

797 Adams, Ruth and Frank Murray. *All you should know about arthritis.* 256pp. 1979. New York: Larchmont Books.

798 Adams, R. and F. Murray. *Beverages: all you should know for your health and well being.* 286pp. 1976. New York: Larchmont Books.

799 Adams, R. and F. Murray. *The good seeds, the rich grains, the hardy nuts, for a healthier, happier life.* 303pp. 1977. New York: Larchmont Books.
Reviews the evidence against refined carbohydrates and discusses the many natural alternatives, their value and uses.

800   Adams, R. and F. Murray. *Health foods.* 342pp. 1983. New York: Larchmont Books.

801   Adams, R. and F. Murray. *Is low blood sugar making you a nutritional cripple?* 174pp. 1983. New York: Larchmont Books.
An excellent review of the literature.

802   Adams, R. and F. Murray. *New high fibre diet.* 319pp. 1980. New York: Larchmont Books.

803   Aihara, Herman. *Acid and alkaline.* 93pp. 1982. Oraville, California: Macrobiotic Foundation.
A classification of health foods into two balancing groups.

804   Airola, Paavo O. *Are you confused?* 222pp. 1981. Phoenix, Arizona: Health Plus.
An excellent introduction to nutrition.

805   Airola, P.O. *Cancer: causes, prevention and treatment.* 40pp. 1972. Phoenix, Arizona: Health Plus.
An excellent overview.

806   Airola, P.O. *Dr. Airola's handbook of natural healing: how to get well.* 303pp. 1983. Phoenix, Arizona: Health Plus.
Presents a complete range of nutritional interventions.

807   Airola, P.O. *Every woman's book: Dr. Airola's practical guide to holistic health.* 638pp. 1982. Phoenix, Arizona: Health Plus.

808   Airola, P.O. *Health secrets from Europe.* 224pp. 1983. New York: Arco. First published in 1970.
An excellent report on the nutrition and vitamin/mineral therapies now in use in Europe.

809   Airola, P.O. *How to keep slim and healthy and young with juice fasting.* 80pp. 1982. Phoenix, Arizona: Health Plus.

810   Airola, P.O. *Hypoglycemia: a better approach.* 191pp. 1981. Phoenix, Arizona: Health Plus.

811   Airola, P.O. *There is a cure for arthritis.* 219pp. 1980. West Nyack, New York: Parker Publishing Company.
Highly recommended.

812   Alexander, Dan Dale. *Arthritis and common sense*. 255pp. 1981. New York: Simon and Schuster.
   Simple dietary advice.

813   Alexander, D.D. *Dry skin and common sense*. 255pp. 1981. New York: Simon and Schuster.
   Simple dietary advice.

814   Alsaker, Rasmus L. *Conquering colds and sinus infections*. 128pp. n.d. New York: Manor Books.

815   Alsaker, R.L. *Eating for health and efficiency*. 509pp. 1928. New York: Grant Publishing Co.

816   Altman, Nathaniel. *Eating for life*. 142pp. 1972. Wheaton, Illinois: Theosophical Publishing House.
   The best single book on vegetarianism.

817   American College of Mechano-therapy. *Clinical lectures*. 476pp. 1912. Chicago, Illinois: American College of Mechano-therapy.
   Lectures on natural cures.

818   American College of Mechano-therapy. *Clinical lecture supplement*. 128pp. 1915. Chicago, Illinois: American College of Mechano-therapy.
   Looks at natural cures for many conditions.

819   Anderson, James W. *Diabetes: a practical new guide to health*. 158pp. 1982. New York: Arco.
   A general overview with an emphasis on diet.

820   Andrews, Gillian (editor). *Bronchitis and emphysema*. 47pp. 1982. Aylesbury, Buckinghamshire: Rodale.

821   Andrews, G. (editor). *Colds and influenza*. 48pp. 1982. Aylesbury, Buckinghamshire: Rodale.

822   Ardell, Donald B. *High level wellness: an alternative to doctors, drugs and disease*. 305pp. 1979. New York: Bantam Books. A revised and updated version of the first edition (published in 1977).

823   Armstrong, J.W. *The water of life: a treatise on urine therapy*. 136pp. 1981. Saffron Walden, Essex: Health Science Press.
   Proposes that all diseases can be cured with this therapy.

824   Atkey, Margaret. *Massage in practice for graduate workers*. 115pp.
n.d. London: The Scientific Press.

825   Auckett, Amelia D. *Baby massage: the magic of the loving touch*.
75pp. 1982. Wellingborough, Northamptonshire: Thorsons.

826   Austin, Reginald F.E. *Direct paths to health: clear thinking, correct
eating and backward breathing*. 104pp. 1923. London: C.W. Daniel.

827   Bailey, Covert. *Fit or fat?* 107pp. 1980. London: Pelham. First
published in 1978.

828   Balantine, Rudolf. *Diet and nutrition: a holistic approach*. 634pp.
1982. Honesdale, Pennsylvania: The Himalyan International Institute.
       An in-depth survey. A classic work that looks at the way foods affect
our health.

829   Balfour, Michael (editor). *The health food guide*. 424pp. 1981.
London: Pan Books.
       A general guide to organizations, nutrition, etc.

830   Banik, Allen E. with Carlson Wade. *Water and your health*. 128pp.
1981. New Canaan, Connecticut: Keats.

831   Bardens, Dennis and G. Philip. *How healthy are you? A plan for
better living*. 129pp. 1972. London: Cassandra Publishers.

832   Barkas, Janet. *The vegetable passion*. 224pp. 1975. New York:
Charles Scribners Sons.
       A well researched social history of vegetarianism.

833   Barker, J. Ellis. *Cancer, how it is caused and how it can be treated*.
432pp. 1924. London: John Murray.

834   Barker, J.E. *Cancer, the surgeon and the researcher*. 483pp. 1928.
London: John Murray.
       A personal approach to the disease calling for a reappraisal of its
cause and treatment.

835   Barker, J.E. *Good health and happiness: a new science of health*.
525pp. 1927. London: John Murray.
       Based on Hippocrates' idea that 'nature is the curer of disease'.

836 Barker, J.E. *New lives for old: how to cure the incurable.* 372pp. 1934. London: John Murray.
  Based on cases the author treated.

837 Barker, Lewis M. (editor). *The psychobiology of human food selection.* 280pp. 1982. Chichester, West Sussex: Ellis Horwood.

838 Barnes, Broda O. and Charlotte W. Barnes. *Hope for hypoglycemia: it's not your mind, it's your liver.* 57pp. 1980. Fort Collins, Colorado: Robinson Press.

839 Barnes, B. and L. Galton. *Hypothyroidism: the unsuspected illness.* 250pp. 1976. Conklin, New York: Thomas Crowell Co.
  An important book.

840 Barreau, Claude and P. Salomon. *The manual of natural living.* 222pp. 1979. Wellingborough, Northamptonshire: Thorsons.
  A simple and informative book covering most nature cures.

841 Barton, F. Alexander. *Good health: How to obtain and maintain it.* 154pp. 1930. London: C.W. Daniel.
  Includes water treatment and dietary therapy.

842 Barton, T. *Nature's plan for your health.* 245pp. 1975. Poole, Dorset: Blandford Press.
  Nature cure and herbal medicine with special reference to cancer, allergies and back pain.

843 Bassler, Thomas and Robert E. Burger. *The whole life diet: an integrated program of nutrition and exercise for a lifestyle of total health.* 203pp. 1979. New York: M. Evans and Co.
  A commonsense approach to fitness and health.

844 Bates, William Horatio. *The Bates method for good sight without glasses.* 159pp. 1944. London: Faber and Faber.
  A new and revised edition of *The cure of imperfect sight by treatment without glasses.*

845 Bates, W.H. *Better eyesight without glasses.* 175pp. 1975. New York: Pyramid Publications.
  A classic.

846   Bates, W.H. *The cure of imperfect sight by treatment without glasses.* 314pp. 1925. New York: Central Fixation Publishing Co. First published in 1920.
The philosophy, theory and practice of the Bates method.

847   Bayley, M. Beddow. *Diet in relation to disease: the case for vegetarianism.* 24pp. n.d. London: The Vegetarian Society.
The Arnold F. Hills Memorial Lecture for 1936.

848   Bazan, W.G. *Healing hands, the drugless profession in America: massage.* 104pp. 1955. Privately published by author.

849   Beck, B.F. and Doree Smedley. *Honey for your health: a nutritional, medical and historical commentary.* 231pp. 1947. London: Museum Press.

850   Benjamin, Harry. *Adventure in living: the autobiography of a myope.* 192pp. 1950. London: Health for All.

851   Benjamin, H. *Better sight without glasses.* 123pp. 1977. Wellingborough, Northamptonshire: Thorsons. First published in 1929.
Diet, exercises, treatments of eye disorders.

852   Benjamin, H. *Common sense vegetarianism.* 64pp. 1981. Wellingborough, Northamptonshire: Thorsons.
Discusses the facts and fictions of the vegetarian diet.

853   Benjamin, H. *Everybody's guide to nature cure.* 481pp. 1983. Wellingborough, Northamptonshire: Thorsons.
A complete guide to the principles of naturopathy.

854   Benjamin, H. *Face living squarely.* 125pp. 1950. London: Health For All.
A 'nature cure' approach to life.

855   Benjamin, H. *Unorthodox healing versus medical science.* 192pp. 1951. London: Health For All.

856   Benjamin, H. *Your diet—in health and disease.* 160pp. 1931. London: Health For All.

857   Berkley, George E. *Cancer: how to prevent it and how to help your doctor fight it.* 242pp. 1978. Englewood Cliffs, New Jersey: Prentice-Hall.
Presents evidence linking cancer to nutrition.

858   Bethel, May. *The healing power of natural foods.* 207pp. 1978.
North Hollywood, California: Wilshire Book Company.

859   Bicknell, Franklin. *Chemicals in food and farm produce: their harmful effects.* 192pp. 1960. London: Faber and Faber.

860   Bieler, Henry G. *Dr. Bieler's natural way to sexual health.* 232pp.
1972. New York: Bantam Books.

861   Bieler, H.G. *Food is your best medicine.* 236pp. 1983. New York:
Ballantine Books.
   A popular book.

862   Binding, G.J. *About pollen: health food and healing agent.* 64pp.
1982. Wellingborough, Northamptonshire: Thorsons.

863   Binding, G.J. *About soya beans.* 96pp. 1970. Wellingborough,
Northamptonshire: Thorsons.

864   Binding, G.J. and Alan Moyle. *About kelp: seaweed for health and vitality.* 63pp. 1979. Wellingborough, Northamptonshire: Thorsons.

865   Bingham, S. *Nutrition.* 383pp. 1978. London: Corgi.
   Discusses better health through good diet.

866   Bircher, Ruth Kunz. *The Bircher-Benner health guide.* 164pp. 1983.
London: Unwin.
   Summarizes the approach to healing of the author's father, Max
Bircher-Benner.

867   Bircher, R. (editor). *Dr. Bircher-Benner's way to positive health and vitality 1867–1967.* 63pp. 1967. Erlenbach–Zürich: Bircher-Benner
Verlag.
   Essays on the centenary of Bircher-Benner's birth.

868   Bircher-Benner, Max. *Children's diet.* 66pp. 1964. London: C.W.
Daniel.
   A practical and theoretical discussion.

869   Bircher-Benner, M. (translated by Arnold Eiloart). *Food science for all and a new sunlight theory of nutrition: lectures to teachers of domestic economy.* 140pp. 1939. London: C.W. Daniel.

870   Bircher-Benner, M. *Health-giving dishes compiled by Bertha Brupbacher-Benner.* 239pp. 1934. London: Edward Arnold.

871   Bircher-Benner, M. *The hell of ill health.* 128pp. 1940. London: John Miles.

872   Bircher-Benner, M. *Liver and gallbladder problems.* 103pp. 1972. Plainview, New York: Nash Publishing Corporation.

873   Bircher-Benner, M. *Nutrition plan for high blood-pressure problems.* 126pp. 1973. New York: Pyramid Publications.

874   Bircher-Benner, M. *Nutrition plan for prostate problems.* 105pp. 1973. Plainview, New York: Nash Publishing Corporation.

875   Bircher-Benner, M. *Nutrition plan for raw food and juices.* 63pp. 1972. Plainview, New York: Nash Publishing Corporation.
    First published in 1959.

876   Bircher-Benner, M. *The prevention of incurable disease.* 128pp. 1981. Cambridge: James Clarke.
    A reprint of the author's seminal work on faulty nutrition.

877   Bircher-Benner (by the staff of the Bircher-Benner Clinic). *Bircher-Benner nutrition plan for arthritis and rheumatism.* 127pp. 1972. New York: Pyramid Publications.

878   Bircher-Benner (by the staff of the Bircher-Benner Clinic). *Nutrition plan for digestive problems.* 142pp. 1971. Plainview, New York: Nash Publishing Corporation.

879   Bircher-Benner (by the staff of the Bircher-Benner Clinic). *Nutrition plan for skin problems.* 124pp. 1977. New York: Pyramid Publications.

880   Bircher-Benner (by the staff of the Bircher-Benner Clinic). *Salt-free nutrition.* 132pp. 1967. Plainview, New York: Nash Publishing Corporation.

881   Bishop, Grace M. *You and your food.* 45pp. 1939. London: C.W. Daniel.
    Dedicated 'to the woman in the home upon whom our health as a nation so largely depends'.

882 Blaine, T.R. *Mental health through nutrition.* 203pp. 1969. Secaucus, New Jersey: Citadel Press.

883 Bland, Jeffrey. *Digestive enzymes: 20 million Americans suffer from digestive orders, are you one of them?* 24pp. 1983. New Canaan, Connecticut: Keats.

884 Bland, J. *Your health under siege: using nutrition to fight back.* 296pp. 1982. Brattleboro, Vermont: The Stephen Greene Press.
Suggests a simple programme of diet, exercise and stress control to reduce the risk of cancer, heart disease and diabetes.

885 Bland, J. *Your personal health programme.* 384pp. 1984. Wellingborough, Northamptonshire: Thorsons.

886 Blumfield, Arthur. *Heart attack: are you a candidate?* 349pp. 1976. New York: Pyramid Publications.

887 Bord, Janet. *Honey: natural food and healer.* 96pp. 1983. Melbourne, Victoria: Science of Life Books.

888 Brady, Margaret. *Children's health and happiness.* 223pp. 1971. Croydon, Surrey: Health For All.

889 Bragg, Paul C. *The miracle of fasting.* 191pp. 1967. Sydney, New South Wales: Health Science Press.
One of Bragg's most popular books on fasting.

890 Brandt, Johanna. *The grape cure for cancer and other diseases.* 168pp. n.d. Dobbes Ferry, New York: Ehret Literature Publishing Corporation. First published in 1928.

891 Brennan, R.O. *Nutrigenetics: a new concept for relieving hypoglycemia.* 257pp. 1975. New York: M. Evans and Company.
Argues the case for better nutrition in preventive medicine.

892 Brewer, Gail and Tom Brewer. *What every pregnant woman should know: the truth about diet and drugs in pregnancy.* 239pp. 1983. Harmondsworth, Middlesex: Penguin.

893 Bricklin, Mark. *The practical encyclopaedia of natural health.* 544pp. 1984. Emmaus, Pennsylvania: Rodale.
Over 120 entries on every aspect of natural health and healing.

894   Brodsky, Greg. *From Eden to Aquarius: The book of natural healing*. 333pp. 1974. New York: Bantam Books.
   A comprehensive guide to nature cure.

895   Brody, Jane. *Jane Brody's nutrition book: a lifetime guide to good eating for better health and weight control*. 552pp. 1982. New York: Bantam Books.
   Popular in America.

896   Bronfen, Nan. *Nutrition for a better life: a source book for the eighties*. 195pp. 1980. Santa Barbara, California: Capra Press.

897   Brown, H.R. *The fast way to health and vigour*. 134pp. 1961. London: Thorsons.

898   Bruder, Roy. *Discovering natural foods*. 292pp. 1982. Santa Barbara, California: Woodbridge Press.

899   Buchinger, Otto H.F. *About fasting: a royal road to healing*. 64pp. 1971. London: Thorsons. First published in 1961.

900   Budd, Martin. *Diets to help diabetes*. 62pp. 1983. Wellingborough, Northamptonshire: Thorsons.

901   Budd, M. *Low blood sugar (hypoglycaemia): the 20th century epidemic?* 127pp. 1982. Wellingborough, Northamptonshire: Thorsons.

902   Burkitt, Denis. *Don't forget fibre in your diet, to help avoid many of our commonest diseases*. 126pp. 1979. London: Martin Dunitz.

903   Burtis, C. Edward. *Nature's miracle medicine chest. How to achieve abundant good health through everyday wonder foods: pure natural foods, our gift from the land and sea*. 170pp. 1974. New York: Arco.

904   Caldwell, Gladys and Philip ZenFagna. *Fluoridation and truth decay*. 301pp. 1974. La Crescenta, California: Top-Ecol Press.
   A well documented study of the dangers of fluoridation.

905   Callow, A. Barbara. *Food and health: an introduction to the study of diet*. 96pp. 1928. London: Oxford University Press.
   For the student and general reader.

906   Cambell, Giraud W. *A doctor's proven new home cure for arthritis*. 224pp. 1984. Wellingborough, Northamptonshire: Thorsons.

907   Carque, Otto. *The key to rational dietetics: Fundamental facts about the prevention of disease. The preservation of health. The prolongation of life.* 151pp. 1930. Los Angeles, California: By author.

908   Carque, O. *Natural foods: the safe way to health.* 359pp. Los Angeles, California: Carque Pure Food Co.

909   Carrington, Hereward. *Fasting for health and long life.* 150pp. 1963. Pasadena, California: Health Research.

910   Carrington, H. *Save your life by fasting.* 226pp. 1969. St. Catherine's, Ontario: Provoker Press.
      A reprint of a pre-World War II book by one of the best-known early hygienists.

911   Carrington, H. *Vitality, fasting and nutrition. A physiological study of the curative power of fasting, together with a new theory of the relations of food to human vitality.* 648pp. 1908. London: Rebman.

912   Carroll, David. *The complete book of natural medicine.* 414pp. 1980. New York: Simon and Schuster.
      Recommended.

913   Cartland, Barbara. *The magic of honey.* 141pp. 1983. London: Corgi.

914   Cerney, J.V. *Modern magic of natural healing with water therapy.* 216pp. 1977. West Nyack, New York: Parker Publishing Company.

915   Chaitow, Boris. *My healing secrets.* 121pp. 1980. Holsworthy, Devon: Health Science Press.
      The philosophy of naturopathy and healthy nutrition simply described.

916   Chaitow, Leon. *An end to cancer? A nutritional approach to its prevention and control.* 127pp. 1978. Wellingborough, Northamptonshire: Thorsons.

917   Charmine, S. *Complete raw juice therapy.* 128pp. 1982. Wellingborough, Northamptonshire: Thorsons.
      A comprehensive guide.

918   Chen, Philip. *Soybeans for health and longer life.* 178pp. 1973. New Canaan, Connecticut: Keats.
      A good, practical guide.

919   Cheraskin, E. and W.M. Ringsdorf Jnr. *New Hope for incurable diseases*. 187pp. 1971. New York: Arco.
An easily understood, concise work.

920   Cheraskin, E., W. M. Ringsdorf Jnr. and Arlie Brecher. *Psychodietics: Food as the key to emotional health*. 239pp. 1981. New York: Bantam Books.
A valid and useful approach to expanding the horizons of people working in mental health settings.

921   Cheraskin, E., W.M. Ringsdorf Jnr. and J.W. Clark. *Diet and disease*. 369pp. 1977. New Canaan, Connecticut: Keats.
One of the best books in the field.

922   Christopher, John R. *Dr. Christopher's three day cleansing program and mucusless diet*. 28pp. 1978. Springville, Utah: Dr. John Christopher.
A detailed collection of dietary and healing instructions.

923   Clark, L. *Get well naturally*. 406pp. 1982. New York: Arco.
A well written, informative survey.

924   Clark, L. *Know your nutrition*. 267pp. 1981. New Canaan, Connecticut: Keats.
A comprehensive book.

925   Clark, L. *Light on your health problems*. 127pp. 1972. New Canaan: Connecticut: Keats.
Question-and-answer format. Looks at additives, diet, vitamins, etc.

926   Clark, L. *Linda Clark's Handbook of natural remedies for common ailments*. 223pp. 1982. Wellingborough, Northamptonshire: Thorsons.
A well organized compendium of healing hints.

927   Clark, L. *The new way to eat*. 174pp. 1980. Millbrae, California: Celestial Arts.
An overview.

928   Clark, L. *Stay younger longer: how to add years of enjoyment to your life*. 396pp. 1961. New York: Pyramid Publications.

929   Clements, G.R. *The law of life and human health.* 1972. Mokelumne Hill, California: Health Research.

930   Clements, Harry. *Arthritis.* 64pp. 1973. Wellingborough, Northamptonshire: Thorsons.

931   Clements, H. *Banishing backaches and disc troubles.* 64pp. 1983. Wellingborough, Northamptonshire: Thorsons.

932   Clements, H. *The causes and treatment of headaches and migraine.* 64pp. 1982. Wellingborough, Northamptonshire: Thorsons.

933   Clements, H. *Diets to help kidney disorders.* 48pp. 1981. Wellingborough, Northamptonshire: Thorsons.

934   Clements, H. *Diets to help prostate troubles.* 48pp. 1980. Wellingborough, Northamptonshire: Thorsons.

935   Clements, H. *Diets to help psoriasis.* 48pp. 1983. Wellingborough, Northamptonshire: Thorsons.

936   Clements, H. *How to save your heart.* 95pp. 1970. London: Thorsons.

937   Clements, H. *Nature cure for painful joints.* 64pp. 1980. Wellingborough, Northamptonshire: Thorsons.

938   Clements, H. *Nature cure for prostate troubles.* 64pp. 1981. Wellingborough, Northamptonshire: Thorsons.

939   Clements, H. *Nature cure for shingles and cold sores.* 64pp. 1979. Wellingborough, Northamptonshire: Thorsons.

940   Clements, H. *The rational treatment of enlarged tonsils and adenoids.* 123pp. 1936. London: Health For All.

941   Clements, H. *Save your tonsils.* 63pp. 1974. Wellingborough, Northamptonshire: Thorsons.

942   Clements, H. *Self-treatment for colitis.* 62pp. 1982. Wellingborough, Northamptonshire: Thorsons.

943   Clements, H. *Self-treatment for hernia.* 63pp. 1979. Wellingborough, Northamptonshire: Thorsons.

944   Clements, H. *Self-treatment for skin troubles.* 64pp. 1983. Wellingborough, Northamptonshire: Thorsons.

945   Clements, H. *Stopping fatigue before it leads to ill health.* 64pp. 1978. Wellingborough, Northamptonshire: Thorsons.

946   Clinkard, C.E. *Eating for health.* 32pp. 1980. London: Whitcoulls Publishers.
      A concise guide.

947   Clymer, R. Swinburne. *Diet a key to health: a series of lessons in the selection and combination of foods for the prevention or cure of disease.* 282pp. 1930. Quakertown, Pennsylvania: The Humanitarian Society.

948   Clymer, R.S. *Making health certain.* 1921. Quakertown, Pennsylvania: The Humanitarian Society.

949   Clymer, R.S. *The natura physician.* 1933. Quakertown, Pennsylvania: Philosophical Publishing Co.

950   Colby, Benjamin. *Guide to health: the Thomsonian system of natural medicine.* 181pp. n.d. Orem, Utah: BiWorld.

951   Committee of Inquiry into Chiropractic, Osteopathy, Homoeopathy and Naturopathy. *Report of the Committee of Inquiry into Chiropractic, Osteopathy, Homoeopathy and Naturopathy.* 925pp. 1977. Canberra, Australia: Australian Government Publishing Service.
      Looks at alternative health care in Australia.

952   Committee on Diet, Nutrition and Cancer; Assembly of Life Sciences; National Research Council. *Diet, nutrition and cancer.* Pages not numbered. 1982. Washington, D.C.: National Academy Press.

953   Copestake, Beatrice M. Goodall. *The theory and practice of massage.* 287pp. 1926. London: H.K. Lewis.
      A comprehensive account.

954   Corbett, Margaret. *How to improve your sight.* 94pp. 1953. New York: Crown Publishers.
      Exercises based on the Bates method.

955   Corbin, Cheryl. *Nutrition: a preventive medicine? Strang Clinic health action plan.* 178pp. 1980. New York: Holt, Rinehart and Winston.
      Shows how to assess your diet and how to put together a more healthful diet.

956   Cornaro, Luigi. *How to live to 100 years.* 93pp. 1951. London: Thorsons.
A reprint of Cornaro's (sixteenth-century Italian nobleman) account of his dietary discoveries.

957   Cott, Allan. *Fasting: the ultimate diet.* 148pp. 1981. New York: Bantam Books.
Putting the case for fasting. Aimed at sceptical medical doctors.

958   Cott, A. *Fasting as a way of life.* 130pp. 1981. New York: Bantam Books.
Geared to the general reader. Intended as a complement to *Fasting: the ultimate diet.*

959   Crook, William G. *Are you allergic?* 166pp. 1978. Jackson, Tennessee: Professional Books.

960   Crook, W.G. *The yeast connection: a medical breakthrough.* 280pp. 1983. Jackson, Tennessee: Professional Books.
Written for the public and the professional.

961   Cureton, T.K. *The physiological effects of wheat germ oils on humans.* 1972. Springfield, Illinois: Charles C. Thomas.

962   Daglish, W.E. *Diet, massage and hydrotherapy.* 1961. Mokelumne Hill, California: Health Research.

963   Dane, Victor. *Grow old, stay young.* 98pp. 1930. London: C.W. Daniel.

964   Daniel, Florence. *Food remedies: facts about foods and their medicinal uses.* 104pp. 1916. London: C. W. Daniel.

965   Darrigol, Jean-Luc. *Cereals for your health: how to benefit from organically grown whole grain cereals.* 128pp. 1984. Wellingborough, Northamptonshire: Thorsons.
A practical guide.

966   Davis, Adelle. *Let's eat right to keep fit.* 303pp. 1984. London: Unwin.
A basic book which contains a lot of useful information.

967   Davis, A. *Let's get well.* 454pp. 1983. London: Unwin.
Recommends dietary principles and practical methods to aid recovery from most common ailments.

968   Davis, A. *Let's have healthy children*. 381pp. 1981. Bergenfield, New Jersey: New American Library.
  A good, practical book.

969   Davis, A. *Let's stay healthy: a guide to lifelong nutrition*. 391pp. 1983. London: Unwin.
  Expert descriptions of what nutrition is, and how it works.

970   Davis, A. *You can get well*. 91pp. 1975. Simi, California: Lust Enterprises.

971   Davison and Passmore. *Human nutrition and dietetics*. 864pp. 1966. Edinburgh: E. and S. Livingstone. First published in 1959.

972   Day, Harvey. *About bread: the controversial cereal*. 64pp. 1973. Wellingborough, Northamptonshire: Thorsons.

973   Day, H. *The breath of life: correct breathing for better health*. 126pp. 1965. London: Thorsons.

974   Deimel, Diana. *Vision victory*. 193pp. 1972. Glendora, California: Diana's Nutrition Center.
  Goes beyond Bates and looks at nutrition, light, homoeopathy, etc., and their effect on eyesight.

975   Densmore, Emmet. *How nature cures: comprising a new system of hygiene and also the natural food of man. A statement of principle arguments against the use of bread, cereals, pulses, potatoes and all other starch foods*. 413pp. 1892. London: Swan Sonnenschein.

976   Dequer, John H. *Health through natural forces*. 255pp. 1924. Los Angeles, California: Grafton Publishing Corporation.

977   Despard, L.L. *Textbook of massage and remedial gymnastics*. 413pp. 1916. London: Published by the joint committees of Henry Frowde, and Hodder and Stoughton.

978   Detmar, Bernherd (translated and edited by Robin Kemball). *Live wisely, live well: an explanation of the value of air, water, sunlight, movement and repose as natural healing factors*. 151pp. 1951. London: Thorsons.

979   De Vries, Arnold. *Therapeutic fasting*. 82pp. 1963. Greone, Iowa: Chandler Book Co.

980   Dewey, Edward Hooker. *The true science of living: the new gospel of health. Practical and physiological. Story of an evolution of natural law in the cure of diseases. For physicians and laymen.* 323pp. 1895. Norwich, Connecticut: The Henry Bill Publishing Co.

981   Dextreit, Raymond (translated and edited by Michael Abehsera). *Our earth, our cure.* 203pp. 1974. New York: Swan House.
Compiled from the forty-three books written by a well-known French naturopath.

982   Dodds, Susanna Way. *Drugless medicine: hygieotherapy.* 1721pp. 1915. London: L.N. Fowler. The Health and Culture Company.
Teaches people how to get well and stay well through hygienic practice and proper diet.

983   Doherty, B. St. John. *Constipation: speedy, complete, permanent cure.* 34pp. 1933. Privately published by author.

984   Doherty, B. St. John. *How to cure goitre by natural methods.* 24pp. 1930. Privately published by author.

985   Doherty, B. St. John. *Rheumatism can be cured.* 46pp. 1933. Privately published by author.
Advocates nature cure.

986   Dole, Lionel. *The blood poisoner.* 80pp. 1965. Croydon, Surrey: Gateway Book Co.
'An exposé of ... vaccination, inoculation and immunization.'

987   Dong, Colin H. and Jane Banks. *New hope for the arthritic.* 248pp. 1983. St. Albans, Hertfordshire: Granada.
Revolves around Dong's diet.

988   DonsBach, K.W. *Preventive organic medicine.* 191pp. 1976. New Canaan, Connecticut: Keats.
A doctor's plan for natural nutrition.

989   Downing, George. *The massage book.* 217pp. 1983. London: Penguin.
One of the first massage books and still one of the best.

990   Downing, G. *Massage and meditation.* 85pp. 1974. Westminster, Maryland: Random House.

991 Dowse, Thomas Stretch. *Lectures on massage and electricity in the treatment of disease.* 447pp. 1906. Bristol, Avon: John Wright.
A textbook for the physician and masseur.

992 Doyle, R. *The vegetarian handbook.* 182pp. 1982. Wellingborough, Northamptonshire: Thorsons.

993 Doyle, Roger and James Redding. *The complete food handbook.* 308pp. 1976. New York: Grove Press.
An excellent reference book.

994 Dufty, William. *Sugar blues.* 255pp. 1975. New York: Warner Books.
A convincing account of the dangers of refined sugar.

995 Duncan, A.H. *About sleep: nature's healing balm.* 62pp. 1970. London: Thorsons.

996 Dunlop, Durham. *The philosophy of the bath, with: a history of hydro-therapeutics and of the hot air bath from the earlier ages.* 465pp. 1873. London: W. Kent.
Of historical interest.

997 Eagle, Robert. *Eating and allergy.* 209pp. 1981. Garden City, New York: Doubleday.

998 Ebbard, Richard J. *Hygiene and self-care: a practical guide for the application of the most efficacious hygienic principles to adults and children, as well as for the radical cure of diseases and chronic diseases based upon modern methods of natural treatment without physic.* 215pp. 1908. London: Modern Medical Publishing Co.

999 Ebner, Maria. *Connective tissue massage: theory and therapeutic application.* 220pp. 1962. London: E. and S. Livingstone.

1000 Ehret, Arnold. *Professor Arnold Ehret's mucusless diet healing system.* 200pp. 1953. Beaumont, California: Ehret Literature Publishing Company.

1001 Ehret, A. *Rational fasting for physical, mental and spiritual rejuvenation.* 87pp. 1975. Beaumont: California: Ehret Literature Publishing Company.

1002 Ehrmantraut, Harry C. *Headaches: the drugless way to lasting relief.* 148pp. 1980. Brookline, Massachusetts: Autumn Press.

1003   Eichenlaub, John. *Home tonics and refreshers for daily health and vigour*. 221pp. 1963. Bergenfield, New Jersey: Award Sales.

1004   Eichenlaub, J. *A Minnesota doctor's home remedies for common and uncommon ailments*. 262pp. 1981. Englewood Cliffs, New Jersey: Prentice-Hall.
   An excellent collection.

1005   Eldricks, Harold, James Crakes and Sam Clarke. *Living longer and better*. 303pp. 1978. Mountain View, California: World Publications.

1006   Elwood, Catherine. *Feel like a million*. 366pp. 1956. New York: Simon and Schuster.
   A good introductory work.

1007   Evans, S.C. *Nutrition in eye health and disease*. 89pp. 1982. London: Roberts Publications.

1008   Faelton, Sharon and the editors of *Prevention* magazine. *The allergy self-help book: A complete guide to detection and natural treatment of allergies*. 320pp. 1984. Emmaus, Pennsylvania: Rodale.
   A useful and practical guide.

1009   Fere, Maud Tresillian. *Does diet cure cancer?* 112pp. 1983. Wellingborough, Northamptonshire: Thorsons.

1010   Fife, John. *Manual of the Turkish bath: heat as a mode of cure and a source of strength for men and animals*. 419pp. 1865. London: John Churchill and Sons.
   From the writings of Mr. Urquhart.

1011   Finkel, Harry. *Health via nature: the health book for the layman. Including a rational system of health, culture and the prevention, treatment and cure of disease by natural methods. Also the study of natural dietetics, the preparation and combination of foods for health and disease*. 270pp. 1925. Los Angeles, California: The Society for Public Health Education.

1012   Flath, Carl. *The miracle nutrient*. 169pp. 1975. New York: Bantam Books.
   A good general book on bowel health.

1013   Forbes, Alec. *The Bristol diet*. 160pp. 1984. London: Century Publishing Company.

Outlines a simple diet designed to remove poisons from the body
and thus help the body avoid or reverse stress diseases.

1014   Fredericks, Carlton. *Eating right for you*. 310pp. 1974. London:
George Allen and Unwin.

1015   Fredericks, C. *Eat well, get well, stay well*. 202pp. 1980. New
York: Grosset and Dunlap.
The latest collection of Dr. Fredericks' nutritional suggestions.

1016   Fredericks, C. *High-fiber way to total health*. 208pp. 1976. New
York: Simon and Schuster.

1017   Fredericks, C. *Look younger, feel healthier*. 310pp. 1972. New
York: Grosset and Dunlap.
Recommended.

1018   Fredericks, C. *New and complete nutrition handbook: your key to good
health*. 272pp. 1979. Huntington Beach, California: The International
Institute of Natural Health Science, Inc.

1019   Fredericks, C. *Psychonutrition*. 224pp. 1976. New York: Grosset
and Dunlap.

1020   Fredericks, C. *Winning the fight against breast cancer: the nutritional
approach*. 208pp. 1977. New York: Grosset and Dunlap.

1021   Fredericks, C. and Herbert Bailey. *Food facts and fallacies*.
380pp. 1978. New York: Arco.
Covers a wide range of subjects.

1022   Fredericks, C. and Herman Goodman. *Low blood sugar, and you*.
1983. New York: The Berkley Publishing Group.
Well written and detailed. Suitable for an educated layman or a
doctor.

1023   Freydberg, Nicholas and W. Gortner. *The food additives book*.
720pp. 1982. New York: Bantam Books.

1024   Frompovich, Catherine, J. *Attacking hay fever and winning!* 27pp.
1981. Coopersburg, Pennsylvania: C.J. Frompovich Publications.

1025   Froude, Charles C. *Right food the right remedy*. 301pp. 1927.
London: Methuen. First published in 1924.

1026   Fuller, Richard R. *Constipation control: an exercise program to achieve regularity*. 43pp. 1981. Smithtown, New York: Exposition Press.

1027   Garten, M.O. *The health secrets of a naturopathic doctor*. 238pp. 1967. Englewood Cliffs, New Jersey: Prentice-Hall.
   A good, clear layman's guide to naturopathy.

1028   Gauquelin, Michael. *How atmospheric conditions affect your health*. 188pp. 1971. New York: ASI.

1029   Gehman, Jesse Mercer. *Living today for tomorrow*. 104pp. 1944. Palerson, New Jersey: Beoma Publishing House.
   About naturopathy and physical culture. Advocates natural healing.

1030   Germann, Donald R. with Margaret Danbrot. *The anti-cancer diet*. 305p. 1977. New York: Peter H. Wyden.

1031   Gerson, Max. *A cancer therapy: results of 50 cases*. 432pp. 1977. Delmar, California: Totality Books.
   A detailed technical book.

1032   Given, D.H. *A new angle on health (nature's provision for the health and happiness of mankind)*. 158pp. 1935. London: John Bale, Sons and Danielsson.
   An introduction to the elementary principles of healthy living.

1033   Glass, Justine. *Nature's way to health*. 158pp. 1972. London: Mayflower Books.
   A good guide to diet and nutrition.

1034   Golstein, J. *Triumph over disease by fasting and natural diet*. 245pp. 1980. New York: Arco.

1035   Gosling, Nalda. *Diets to help gall bladder troubles*. 48pp. 1980. Wellingborough, Northamptonshire: Thorsons.

1036   Graham, J. *Multiple sclerosis: A self help guide to its management*. 167pp. 1982. Wellingborough, Northamptonshire: Thorsons.

1037   Graham, Sylvester, Russell T. Trall, Herbert M. Shelton and others. *The greatest health discovery: natural hygiene and its evolution past, present and future*. 241pp. 1972. Chicago, Illinois: Natural Hygiene Press.

A book of readings, including nineteenth-century writings, with commentary.

1038 Grainger, Noice B. *Practical nature cure without drugs.* 128pp. 1924. London: C.W. Daniel.

1039 Grant, Doris. *Fluoridation and the forgotten issue: a personal submission to the Prime Minister.* 60pp. n.d. Thames Ditton, Surrey: National Anti-Fluoridation Compaign.

1040 Grant, D. *Your bread and your life.* 243pp. 1961. London: Faber and Faber.
Discusses the dangers of factory-produced bread.

1041 Grant, D. *Your daily food: recipe for survival.* 207pp. 1974. London: Faber and Faber.
Demonstrates how modern man's mode of life is related to modern diseases and how we can reduce the damage.

1042 Grant, D. and Jean Joice. *Food combining for health.* 240pp. 1984. Wellingborough, Northamptonshire: Thorsons.

1043 Gray, Robert. *The colon health handbook: new health through colon rejuvenation.* 76pp. 1983. Oakland, California: Rockridge Publishing Company.

1044 Greer, J.H. *A physician in the house for family and individual consultation.* 956pp. 1930. Chicago, Illinois: Max Stein Publishing Company.
Still an important work for naturopaths. Includes rules for healthy living, disease and treatment.

1045 Greer, Rita. *Diets to help multiple sclerosis.* 47pp. 1982. Wellingborough, Northamptonshire: Thorsons.

1046 Greer, R. and Robert Woodward. *Food allergy: a practical, easy guide.* 80pp. 1982. London: Roberts Publications.

1047 Haas, Elson M. *Staying healthy with the seasons.* 242pp. 1981. Millbrae, California: Celestial Arts.

1048 Haffer, Jack. *Total massage.* 223pp. 1976. New York: Grosset and Dunlap.

1049   Hall, George. *Healthy feet*. 62pp. 1973. Wellingborough, Northamptonshire: Thorsons.

1050   Hall, G. *How to banish colds and influenza*. 64pp. 1982. Wellingborough, Northamptonshire: Thorsons.
   Suggestions of natural treatments.

1051   Hall, G. *How to overcome anaemia*. 64pp. 1977. Wellingborough, Northamptonshire: Thorsons.

1052   Hall, Ross. *Food for nought: the decline in nutrition*. 324pp. 1976. Westminster, Maryland: Random House.
   A well documented technical survey.

1053   Hanssen, Maurice. *About the salt of life*. 96pp. 1982. Wellingborough, Northamptonshire: Thorsons. First published in 1968.

1054   Hanssen, M. *Hanssen's complete cider vinegar*. 128pp. 1983. Wellingborough, Northamptonshire: Thorsons.

1055   Hanssen, M. *Healing power of pollen and other products from the bee hive (propolis, royal jelly, honey)*. 95pp. 1982. Wellingborough, Northamptonshire: Thorsons.

1056   Hanssen, M. and Jack Eden. *Natural cold cures: safe and effective remedies for beating and treating the common cold*. 64pp. 1979. Wellingborough, Northamptonshire: Thorsons.

1057   Hare, Francis. *The food factor in disease*. 2 volumes. 1906. London: Longmans, Greens and Co. First published in 1905.

1058   Harris, Ben Charles. *Kitchen medicines*. 174pp. 1961. New York: Simon and Schuster.
   An interesting reference book.

1059   Harris, John F. *Swedish massage: a systematic and practical approach*. 107pp. 1983. Romford, Essex: L. N. Fowler.

1060   Haught, S. J. *Has Dr. Max Gerson a true cancer cure?* 160pp. 1967. North Hollywood, California: London Press.
   A fascinating account.

1061   Hauser, Benjamin Gayelord. *Be happier, be healthier*. 287pp. 1953. London: Faber and Faber.

Suggests that health depends on sun, air, earth, water and green things.

1062   Hauser, B.G. *Better eyesight without glasses*. 80pp. 1962. London: Faber and Faber. First published in 1942.
Diets, exercises, vitamins, etc.

1063   Hauser, B.G. *Dictionary of foods*. 135pp. 1970. Simi, California: Lust Enterprises.

1064   Hauser, B.G. *Gayelord Hauser's new treasury of secrets*. 425pp. 1974. London: Faber and Faber.
A comprehensive look at naturopathy.

1065   Hauser, B.G. *Harmonized food selection: including the famous Hauser body building system*. 120pp. 1930. New York: Tempo Books.

1066   Hauser, B.G. *Look younger, live longer*. 320pp. 1951. London: Faber and Faber.
Contains mostly diets.

1067   Hawksey, H. *Cider apple vinegar: explains the restorative powers of this unique folk remedy*. 48pp. 1983. Melbourne, Victoria: Science of Life Books.

1068   Hawksey, H. *Get well with food*. 64pp. 1976. Wellingborough, Northamptonshire: Thorsons.

1069   Hawschka, Rudolf (translated by Marjorie Spock and Mary T. Richards). *Nutrition*. 212pp. 1967. London: Stuart and Watkins.

1070   Hay, William Howard (edited by F.A. Robinson). *Building better bodies*. 190pp. 1936. London: George G. Harrap.
Nutrition and health.

1071   Hay, W.H. (edited by Rasmus Alsaker). *Health via food*. 317pp. 1934. London, George G. Harrap.

1072   Hayhurst, Emery R. *Personal health*. 279pp. 1927. New York: McGraw-Hill.
A practical health guide.

1073   Hazzard, Linda Burfield. *Scientific fasting*. 1963. Mokelumne Hill, California: Health Research.

1074   Heinerman, John. *Aloe vera, jojoba and yucca: the amazing health benefits they can give you.* 25pp. 1982. New Canaan, Connecticut: Keats.

1075   Heinl, Tina. *The baby massage book.* 62pp. 1982. London: Coventure.
   Beautifully illustrated.

1076   Hewlett-Parsons, J. *ABC of nature cure.* 192pp. 1968. New York: Arco.
   A good overall introduction to naturopathy.

1077   Hewlett-Parsons, J. *Naturopathic practice: a textbook.* 192pp. 1968. London: Thorsons.

1078   Hightower, Jim. *Eat your heart out: how food profiteers victimize the consumer.* 294pp. 1974. Westminster, Maryland: Random House.
   A well written technical study.

1079   Hill, Ray. *Bran and other natural aids to intestinal fitness.* 64pp. 1979. Wellingborough, Northamptonshire: Thorsons.
   An introductory discussion.

1080   Hills, Christopher. *The secrets of spirulina.* 218pp. 1980. Boulder Creek, California: University of the Trees Press.
   A collection of research reports by Japanese scientists and physicians.

1081   Hills, Hilda Cherry. *Good food, gluten free.* 178pp. 1976. London: Robert Publications.
   Includes descriptions of coeliac disease and other illnesses that may result from gluten.

1082   Hindhede, Mikkel. *Protein and nutrition: an investigation.* 201pp. 1915. London: Ewart Seymour and Co.

1083   Hoffer, Abram and Morton Walker. *Nutrients to age without senility.* 230pp. 1980. New Canaan, Connecticut: Keats.
   Suggests that senility is a form of malnutrition and can be avoided, even reversed, by sound nutritional planning and therapy.

1084   Hoffman, Frederick L. *Cancer and diet: with facts and observations on related subjects.* 767pp. 1937. Baltimore: The Williams and Wilkins Company.

1085   Holford, Patrick. *The whole health manual: the comprehensive guide to nutrition and better health*. 114pp. 1983. Wellingborough, Northamptonshire: Thorsons.

1086   Homola, Samuel. *Dr. Homola's life-extender health guide*. 223pp. 1975. Englewood Cliffs, New Jersey: Prentice-Hall.

1087   Homola, S. *Dr. Homola's natural health remedies*. 250pp. 1973. Englewood Cliffs, New Jersey: Prentice-Hall.

1088   Howard, Alan N. and I. McLean Baird (editors). *Nutritional deficiencies in modern society*. 109pp. 1973. London: Newman Books.

1089   Howell, Edward. *Food enzymes for health and longevity*. 124pp. 1980. Woodsrock Valley, Connecticut: Omangod Press.

1090   Hulbert, H.H. *Natural physical remedies: light, heat, electricity and exercise in the treatment of disease*. 267pp. 1903. London: Simpkin, Marshall, Hamilton, Kent and Co.
        The outcome of long and careful investigation.

1091   Hunt, J. *Raw food way to health: change your eating habits and change your life*. 95pp. 1978. Wellingborough, Northamptonshire: Thorsons.
        A convincing argument for a diet mostly of raw foods.

1092   Hunter, Beatrice Trum. *Additives book: what you need to know*. 136pp. 1980. New Canaan, Connecticut: Keats.

1093   Hunter, B.T. *Brewer's yeast, wheat germ and other high power foods: the foods that enrich you nutritionally ... what you need to know*. 26pp. 1982. New Canaan, Connecticut: Keats.

1094   Hunter, B.T. *Consumers beware! Your food and what's been done to it*. 431pp. 1976. New York: Simon and Schuster.
        Recommended.

1095   Hunter, B.T. *Fact book on fermented foods and beverages*. 116pp. 1973. New Canaan, Connecticut: Keats.
        A useful guide.

1096   Hunter, B.T. *Fact book on yogurt, Kefir and other milk cultures*. 117pp. 1973. New Canaan, Connecticut: Keats.

1097   Hunter, B.T. *The natural foods primer: help for the bewildered beginner.* 119pp. 1979. London: Unwin.
A good practical guide.

1098   Hunter, B.T. *Wheat, millet and other grains: the 'nutritional storehouses' and their health benefits.* 26pp. 1982. New Canaan, Connecticut: Keats.

1099   Hunter, Lorraine. *The vital nutrient counter.* 80pp. 1980. St. Albans, Hertfordshire: Granada.
Looks at the nutrient breakdown of a variety of foods.

1100   Hur, Robin. *Food reform: our desperate need.* 264pp. 1975. Colorado, Texas: Heidelberg Press.
A controversial book.

1101   International Health Council. *A program for the prevention, detection and reversal of pre-cancerous conditions.* 44pp. 1974. Cleveland, Ohio: International Health Council.
Recommended as the best brief treatment of the subject.

1102   Irwin, H.M. *An apple a day.* 167pp. n.d. London: Geoffrey L. Rudd.
Natural health and cure.

1103   Irwin, H.M. *Health for ever.* 160pp. n.d. London: Rider.
Fasting and correct diet.

1104   Issels, Joseph. *Cancer: a second opinion.* 216pp. 1975. Sevenoaks, Kent: Hodder and Stoughton.

1105   Jacka, Judy. *Cancer: a physical and psychic profile.* 78pp. 1977. Hawthorn, Victoria: Jacka's Naturopathic Centres.
Covers many naturopathic treatments for cancer.

1106   Jacka, J. *Natural healing.* 6pp. n.d. Hawthorn, Victoria: Jacka's Naturopathic Centres.
A summary of naturopathy.

1107   Jacka, J. *A philosophy of healing.* 94pp. 1979. Melbourne, Victoria: Inkata Press.

1108   Jacka, P.A. *Naturopathic clinical medicine.* 112pp. 1981. Melbourne, Victoria: Southern School of Natural Therapies.
A repertory and guide to prescribing.

1109   Jackson, Jim. *Seeing yourself see.* 125pp. 1975. New York: E. P. Dutton.
Excellent

1110   Jackson, Richard. *Massage therapy: the holistic way to physical and mental health.* 128pp. 1982. Wellingborough, Northamptonshire: Thorsons.

1111   Jackson, Robert G. *I defy disease ... why not you.* 454pp. n.d. Toronto, Ontario: Miln-Bingham Printcraft.
A reconstructed edition of *How to be always well.*

1112   Jacobson, Michael. *Eater's digest.* 260pp. 1972. Garden City, New York: Doubleday.
Good.

1113   James, Don. *Folk and modern medicine.* 320pp. 1961. Derby, Connecticut: Monarch Books.

1114   Jarrett, Bonnie (compiler). *Health by choice: an anthology.* 1984. New Canaan, Connecticut: Keats.
Experts in the field of preventive medicine present their research. A comprehensive survey.

1115   Jarvis, D.C. *Arthritis and folk medicine.* 158pp. 1983. London: Pan Books.
Fascinating and useful reading.

1116   Jarvis, D.C. *Folk medicine: a doctor's guide to good health.* 184pp. 1983. London: Pan Books. First published in 1958.
Contains a great deal of useful information.

1117   Jeans, Helen. *Natural oils from nuts and seeds: their unique cooking and healing properties.* 63pp. 1978. Wellingborough, Northamptonshire: Thorsons.

1118   Jeffery, Clement. *Human powers.* 227pp. 1929. London: Mills and Boon.
Natural Methods which prevent and cure conditions of disease.

1119   Jeffery, C. *Positive health: without knife or drugs.* 132pp. 1928. London: Mills and Boon.

1120   Jenks, Jorian. *The stuff man's made of: the positive approach to health through nutrition.* 246pp. 1959. London: Faber and Faber.

1121   Jensen, B. *Health magic through chlorophyll.* 154pp. 1973. Solana Beach, California: Jensen's Nutritional and Health Products.

1122   Jensen, B. *Overcoming arthritis and rheumatism.* 55pp. n.d. Solana Beach, California: Jensen's Nutritional and Health Products.
A collection of diet suggestions and healing hints.

1123   Jensen, B. *Seeds and sprouts for life.* 50pp. n.d. Solana Beach, California: Jensen's Nutritional and Health Products.
A detailed survey of the medicinal value of seeds and grains.

1124   Jensen, B. *You can master disease: lessons dealing with the causes of disease and how they can be prevented.* 229pp. 1952. Solana Beach, California: Bernard Jensen Publishing Company.

1125   Johnson, Charles W. *Fasting, longevity and immortality.* 218pp. 1978. Haddam, Connecticut: Survival Press.

1126   Kadans, Joseph. *Encyclopaedia of fruits, vegetables, nuts and seeds for healthful living.* 215pp. 1973. Englewood Cliffs, New Jersey: Prentice-Hall.

1127   Kadans, J. *Encyclopaedia of medicinal foods.* 208pp. 1982. Wellingborough, Northamptonshire: Thorsons.

1128   Keller, Jeanne. *Healing with water.* 1968. New York: Award Books.

1129   Kelly, William. *New hope for cancer victims.* 42pp. 1969. Denver, Colorado: Nutri-Books.
An excellent discussion of Kelly's cancer treatment.

1130   Kellogg, John Harvey. *Art of massage.* 1929. Battle Creek, Michigan: Modern Medicine Publishing Co.

1131   Kellogg, J.H. *The crippled colon: causes, consequences, remedies.* 385pp. 1931. Battle Creek, Michigan: Modern Medicine Publishing Co.

1132   Kellogg, J.H. *How to have good health through biologic living.* 498pp. 1932. Battle Creek, Michigan: Modern Medicine Publishing Co.
Diet, sunlight, hygiene.

1133   Kellogg, J.H. *The natural diet of man*. 386pp. 1923. Battle Creek, Michigan: Modern Medicine Publishing Co.

1134   Kelso, Isa Anderson. *The causes and treatment of women's ailments*. 64pp. 1981. Wellingborough, Northamptonshire: Thorsons.

1135   Kenton, Leslie and Susannah Kenton. *Raw energy: eat your way to radiant health*. 256pp. 1984. London: Century.
A well researched book on the benefits of a mainly raw-food diet.

1136   Keough, Carol and the editors of *Prevention* magazine. *Natural relief for arthritis*. 272pp. 1984. Emmaus, Pennsylvania: Rodale.
A helpful guide that offers natural ways to relieve pain.

1137   Kezdi, Paul. *You and your heart: how to take care of your heart for a long and healthy life*. 222pp. 1981. London: Penguin.
Covers diet and relaxation.

1138   Kidman, Brenda. *A gentle way with cancer: what every cancer patient should know about the therapies which can influence the fight for recovery*. 182pp. 1983. London: Century Publishing Company.

1139   Kilmartin, Angela. *Cystitis: a complete self-help guide*. 199pp. 1981. Feltham, Middlesex: Hamlyn Paperbacks.

1140   Kinderlehrer, Jane. *How to feel younger longer*. 220pp. 1974. Emmaus, Pennsylvania: Rodale.
A good discussion of the nutritional aspects of the ailments and diseases of ageing.

1141   Kirk, *Professor* (edited by Edward Bruce Kirk). *Papers on health*. 392pp. 1930. London: Simpkin Marshall, Hamilton, Kent and Co.
Nature cure.

1142   Kirschmann, John D. *Nutrition almanac*. 279pp. 1979. London: McGraw-Hill.
Food nutrition and health questions knowledgeably addressed.

1143   Klen, Emil A.G. (translated by Mina L. Dobbie). *Massage and medical gymnastics*. 618pp. 1918. London: J. and A. Churchill.

1144   Kloss, Jethro. *Back to Eden.* 688pp. 1984. Santa Barbara, California: Woodbridge Press.
The World's best-known health book.

1145   Knagg, H. Valentine. *Consumption and tomorrow.* 36pp. 1926. London: C. W. Daniel.
Nature cure.

1146   Knagg, H.V. *An epitome of the 'nature cure' system of medicine.* 28pp. 1925. London: C.W. Daniel.
A pamphlet.

1147   Knagg, H.V. *Help for chronic sufferers.* 134pp. n.d. London: Jarrold and Sons.

1148   Knagg, H.V. *How to prevent cancer: the story of the origin and growth of cancer. How cancer can be avoided. Necessity for reform of medical research and practice.* 56pp. 1932. London: C.W. Daniel.

1149   Knagg, H.V. *Indigestion: its cause and cure.* 128pp. 1916. London: C. W. Daniel

1150   Knagg, H.V. *The truth about sugar.* 79pp. n.d. London: C. W. Daniel

1151   Kneipp, Sebastian. *My water cure: as tested through more than 30 years and described for the healing diseases and preservation of health.* 272pp. 1901. Edinburgh: William Blackwood. First published in 1893.

1152   Kneipp, S. *Thus shalt thou live: hints and advice for the healthy and the sick on a simple rational mode of life and a natural method of cure.* 389pp. 1905. Kempten, Bavaria, Germany: Jos Koesel.

1153   Kohler, Jean Charles and Mary Alice Kohler. *Healing miracles from macrobiotics.* 292pp. 1979. Englewood Cliffs, New Jersey: Prentice-Hall.

1154   Kordel, Lelord. *Eat your troubles away.* 254pp. 1956. London: Herbert Jenkins.

1155   Kordel, L. *Health through nutrition.* 352pp. 1075. New York: Manor Books.

1156   Kretchmer, N. and W. Robertson. *Human nutrition.* 275pp.

1978. San Francisco, California: W. H. Freeman. First published in 1952.

1157   Kugler, Hans. *Slowing down the aging process*. 236pp. 1975. New York: Pyramid Publications.

1158   Kuhne, Louis. *The new science of healing: or the doctrine of the oneness of all diseases forming a basis of a uniform method of cure without medicines and without operations*. 458pp. 1892. Leipzig, Germany: By author.
An eccentric offshoot of nature cure, 'the Science of Facial Expression'.

1159   Kushi, Michio. *The book of macrobiotics: the universal way of health and happiness*. 182pp. 1981. Tokyo, Japan: Japan Publications. First published in 1977.

1160   Kushi, M. *The macrobiotic approach to cancer: towards preventing and controlling cancer with diet and lifestyle*. 126pp. 1982. Wayne, New Jersey: Avery Publishing Group.

1161   Kushi, M. (edited by Edward Esko). *Natural healing through macrobiotics*. 204pp. 1979. Tokyo, Japan: Japan Publications.

1162   Kushi, M., Edward Esko and Marc Van Cauwenberghe (editors). *The macrobiotic approach to major illnesses*. 1978. Boston, Massachusetts: East–West Foundation.

1163   Kushi, M. and Alex Jack. *The cancer prevention diet: Michio Kushi's nutritional blueprint for the relief and prevention of disease*. 416pp. 1984. Wellingborough, Northamptonshire: Thorsons.
A valuable and up-to-date thesis.

1164   Kushi, M. and others (edited by Edward Esko). *Cancer and heart disease. The macrobiotic approach to degenerative diseases*. 224pp. 1982. Tokyo: Japan Publications.

1165   Kuts-Chereaux, A. *Naturae medicina and naturopathic dispensatory*. 1975. Yellow Springs, Ohio: Antioch Press.
Written by a member of the American Naturopathic Physicians and Surgeons Association.

1166   Lavan, Fay and Jean Dalrymple. *The folklore and facts of natural nutrition*. 190pp. 1974. New York: Arco.

1167   Law, Donald. *You are how you eat.* 220pp. 1977. London: Turnstone Books.

1168   Lawrence, Ronald M. and Stanley Rosenberg. *Pain relief with osteomassage: at your fingertips, a revolutionary and simple new method for relaxation and relief from pain.* 92pp. 1982. Santa Barbara, California: Woodbridge Press.

1169   Lawson-Wood, D. and J. Lawson-Wood. *Glowing health through diet and posture.* 62pp. 1973. Holsworthy, Devon: Health Science Press.
An introduction to Dr. Sekwazawa's teachings on macrobiotic diet.

1170   Lay, Joan. *Diets to help colitis.* 48pp. 1982. Wellingborough, Northamptonshire: Thorsons.

1171   Lay, J. *Self-help for hiatus hernia.* 63pp. 1983. Wellingborough, Northamptonshire: Thorsons.

1172   Leboyer, Fredrick. *Loving hands: the traditional Indian art of baby massage.* 135pp. 1982. New York: Alfred A. Knopf.

1173   Lederman, E.K. *Good health through natural therapy: the common sense guide book to a healthier life.* 147pp. 1978. London: Pan Books.

1174   Lederman, E.K. *Natural therapy: an exposition of the scientific and educational aspects of nature cure.* 180pp. 1953. London: Watts and Co.

1175   Lee, William H. *The book of raw fruit and vegetable juices and drinks.* 177pp. 1982. New Canaan, Connecticut: Keats.

1176   Leibold, Gerhard. *Practical hydrotherapy: a home guide to water cure treatment.* 96pp. 1980. Wellingborough, Northamptonshire: Thorsons.

1177   Leitch, J. Neil. *What to eat and why.* 68pp. 1936. London: London College of Dietetics.
A textbook; of general historical interest.

1178   Leonard, J.N., J.L. Hoper and N. Pritkin. *Live longer now.* 252pp. 1974. New York: Grosset and Dunlap.
A practical guide.

1179   Lewis, Alan. *The Japanese oyster: amazing healing properties from the sea.* 64pp. 1981. Wellingborough, Northamptonshire: Thorsons.

1180   Lief, Stanley. *Diet reform simplified.* 63pp. 1933. London: Health For All.

1181   Lief, S. *How to eat for health.* 96pp. 1979. New York: Baronet Publishing Company. First published in 1933.
   A sensible and logical presentation of the principles of health through diet.

1182   Lief, S. *How to feed children from infancy onwards.* 58pp. 1933. London: Health For All.

1183   Light, Marilyn. *Hypoglycemia: one of man's most widespread and misdiagnosed diseases.* 26pp. 1983. New Canaan, Connecticut: Keats.

1184   Lindlahr, Ann and Henry Lindlahr. *The Lindlahr vegetarian cookbook.* 1922. Chicago, Illinois: Lindlahr Publishing Company.
   A pioneer book.

1185   Lindlahr, Henry. *Natural therapeutics.* Volume 1: *Philosophy of natural therapeutics.* 327pp. 1975. Maidstone, Kent: The Maidstone Osteopathic Clinic. First published in 1926.

1186   Lindlahr, H. *Natural therapeutics.* Volume 2: *Practice of natural therapeutics.* 313pp. 1981. Saffron Walden, Essex: C.W. Daniel. First published in 1919.

1187   Lindlahr, H. *Natural therapeutics.* Volume 3: *Dietetics.* 169pp. 1983. Saffron Walden, Essex: C.W. Daniel.

1188   Lindlahr, H. *Natural therapeutics.* Volume 4: *Iridiagnosis and other diagnostic methods.* 334pp. 1919. Chicago, Illinois: Lindlahr Publishing Co.

1189   Lindlahr, H. *Nature cure: philosophy and practice based on the unity of disease and cure.* 430pp. 1922. Chicago, Illinois: The Nature Cure Publishing Co.

1190   Lindlahr, Victor H. *You are what you eat.* 128pp. 1971. Van Nuys, California: Newcastle Publishing Company.
   How to eat for your health's sake.

1191   Llewellyn-Jones, Derek. *Every body: a nutritional guide to life.* 249pp. 1980. Oxford: Oxford University Press.
   Facts and fallacies about food and disease.

1192   Lloyd, Eileen (editor). *Arthritis*. 46pp. 1982. Aylesbury, Buckinghamshire: Rodale.

1193   Lloyd, E. (editor). *Backache*. 46pp. 1982. Aylesbury, Buckinghamshire: Rodale.

1194   Lloyd, E. (editor). *Cancer risk and your diet*. 45pp. 1982. Aylesbury, Buckinghamshire: Rodale.

1195   Lloyd, E. (editor). *Headaches and migraine*. 47pp. 1982. Aylesbury, Buckinghamshire: Rodale.

1196   Lloyd, E. (editor). *Ulcers*. 46pp. 1982. Aylesbury, Buckinghamshire: Rodale.

1197   Lowe, Carl. *Whole body healing: natural healing with movement, exercise, massage and other drug-free methods*. 576pp. 1984. Emmaus, Pennsylvania: Rodale.

1198   Lowenfield, Clare. *Everything you should know about your food*. 288pp. 1978. London: Faber and Faber.
    A valuable source of information and detailed guidance.

1199   Lucas, J.W. *Vegetarian nutrition*. 136pp. 1979. Altrincham, Cheshire: The Vegetarian Society of The United Kingdom.
    A definitive work on the science of nutrition with vegetarian principles.

1200   Luderman, Kate, Louise Henderson and Henry S. Bassayne. *Do-it-yourself allergy analysis handbook*. 154pp. 1979. New Canaan, Connecticut: Keats.

1201   Luftig, William. *How to cure eye diseases without operation*. 387pp. 1939. London: C.W. Daniel.

1202   Luftig, W. *The natural treatment of eye disease*. 244pp. 1947. London: Health For All.
    Diet, light, colour, etc.

1203   Luftig, W. *Victory over eye diseases without operation: an outline of my system of non-operative treatment*. 128pp. 1940. London: C.W. Daniel.

1204   Lust, John B. *About raw juices: their therapeutical value and uses*. 62pp. 1982. Wellingborough, Northamptonshire: Thorsons.

1205   Lust, J.B. *Drink your troubles away.* 210pp. 1981. New York: Benedict Lust Publications.
An excellent presentation of the argument for raw juice therapy.

1206   Lust, J.B. *Raw juice therapy.* 173pp. 1974. Wellingborough, Northamptonshire: Thorsons.

1207   Lutzner, Hellmut. *The secrets of successful fasting: a day-to-day guide.* 64pp. 1983. Wellingborough, Northamptonshire: Thorsons.

1208   Lyngheim, Linda and Jack Scagnetti. *Bee pollen: nature's miracle health food.* 90pp. 1979. North Hollywood, California: Wilshire Book Company.

1209   McCann, Alfred W. *The science of eating: how to insure stamina, endurance, vigor, strength and health in infancy, youth and age.* 408pp. 1919. Garden City, New York: Garden City Publishing Company.

1210   McCarrison, Robert. *Nutrition and health.* 127pp. 1982. London: McCarrison Society.
First given as a lecture to the Royal Society of Arts in 1936. Also includes two earlier essays.

1211   McCoy, Frank. *The fast way to health, being as to the first part, an exposition of the fasting cure and its application to prevalent disorders, and as to the second part, a treatise on food, together with diets for the well.* 333pp. 1926. Los Angeles, California: McCoy Publications.

1212   McCutcheon, Ralph. *Diets to help cystitis.* 48pp. 1983. Wellingborough, Northamptonshire: Thorsons.

1213   McDonagh, J.E.R. *A further study in the nature of disease.* 372pp. 1954. London: William Heinemann Medical Books.
An unusual and interesting book.

1214   MacFadden, Bernarr. *Eating for health and strength.* 276pp. 1924. New York: MacFadden Publications.

1215   MacFadden, B. *Fasting for health.* 206pp. 1978. New York: Arco.
One of the most authoritative books on the subject.

1216   MacFadden, B. *Headaches: how caused and how cured.* 211pp. 1925. New York: MacFadden Publications.

Views headaches as symptoms of other conditions and suggests natural treatments accordingly.

1217　MacFadden, B. *MacFadden's encyclopaedia of physical culture.* Volume 1: 583pp. Volume 2: 1202pp. Volume 3: 1793pp. Volume 4: 2407pp. Volume 5: 2969pp. 1918. New York: Physical Culture Publishing Company.
A complete system of diet, sun and exercise.

1218　MacFadden, B. *The miracle of milk: how to use the milk diet scientifically at home.* 204pp. 1926. New York: MacFadden Publications.

1219　MacFadden, B. *Natural cure for rupture: a rational, natural means of permanently curing rupture.* 107pp. n.d. Physical Culture Publishing Co. No address given.

1220　MacFadden, B. *Strengthening the eyes: a system of scientific eye training.* 1929. New York: MacFadden Publications.

1221　MacFadden, B. *Vitality supreme.* 259pp. 1915. London: Health For All.
Diet and exercise for a healthy, strong body.

1222　MacFarlane, Helen. *Arthritis: help in your own hands.* 96pp. 1970. London: Thorsons.
Massage, diet, exercise, etc.

1223　MacFarlane, H. *Diets to help arthritis.* 48pp. 1982. Wellingborough, Northamptonshire: Thorsons.

1224　McGarey, William A. *The Edgar Cayce remedies.* 217pp. 1983. New York: Bantam Books.
A practical holistic approach.

1225　McGrath, William. *Bio-nutronics.* 216pp. 1972. Bergenfield, New Jersey: New American Library.
A good general advice book on health and nutrition.

1226　MacKarness, Richard. *Chemical victims.* 203pp. 1983. London: Pan Books.
Discusses the use of nutritional therapy in the place of chemicals and drugs.

1227   McKeon, L.C. Floyd. *A healing crisis*. 175pp. 1933. Weston-super-Mare, Avon: Michell Health Products.
Looks at naturopathy, osteopathy and chiropractic.

1228   McKie, William L. *Scientific hydrotherapy*. 135pp. 1957. Mokelumne Hill, California: Health Research.
Based on a series of lectures given in 1915–16 to students at the American College of Neuropathy in Philadelphia.

1229   MacMickle, Virgil. *Eat and be healthy: the diet question simplified*. 122pp. 1929. London: C. W. Daniel. First published in 1921.

1230   Mae, Eydic with Chris Loeffler. *How I conquered cancer naturally*. 237pp. n.d. Irvine, California: Harvest House.

1231   Mallett, Reddie. *Nature's way: a means of health without medicine*. 46pp. 1930. London: Watts and Co.

1232   Malstrom, Stan. *Own your own body*. 398pp. 1980. New Canaan, Connecticut: Keats.
A comprehensive volume filled with practical information and insights.

1233   Malstrom, S. and Jared Brown. *Your colon: its character, care and therapy*. 34pp. 1981. Orem, Utah: BiWorld.

1234   Mandell, Marshall. *Dr. Mandell's lifetime arthritis relief system*. 271pp. 1983. Toronto, Canada: General Publishing Company.

1235   Mandell, M. and Lynne Waller Scanion. *Dr. Mandell's five day allergy relief system*. 321pp. 1983. London: Arrow Books.

1236   Marsh, E.E. *How to be healthy with natural foods*. 164pp. 1978. New York: Arco.

1237   Maryon-Davis, Alan with Jane Thomas. *Diet 2000*. 128pp. 1984. London: Pan Books.
A practical guide to better nutrition.

1238   Meagher, Jack and Pat Boughton. *Sports massage*. 215pp. 1980. Garden City, New York: Doubleday.
Presents a complete programme for increasing performance and endurance.

1239   Mellor, Constance. *Constance Mellor's natural remedies for common ailments*. 256pp. 1982. London: Granada.

1240   Mellor, C. *Guide to natural health*. 127pp. 1982. London: Granada.

1241   Mennell, James. *Massage: its principles and practice*. 535pp. 1920. London: J. and A. Churchill.

1242   Mervyn, Leonard. *High blood pressure: sound nutritional principles for the control of hypertension by dietary means*. 96pp. 1983. Melbourne, Victoria: Science of Life Books.

1243   Mervyn, L. *Woman's change of life: natural treatments and dietary advice for easing the effects of the menopause*. 96pp. 1983. Melbourne, Victoria: Science of Life Books.

1244   Mességué, Maurice. *Way to natural health and beauty*. 254pp. 1974. New York: Macmillan.
   Contains good practical advice.

1245   Metcalfe, Richard. *Life of Vincent Priessnitz: founder of hydrotherapy*. 210pp. 1898. London: London Hydro.

1246   Metcalfe, R. *The rise and progress of hydrotherapy in England*. 307pp. 1906. London: Simpkin, Marshall, Hamilton, Kent and Co.

1247   Michaels, Marjorie. *Stay healthy with wine: natural cures and beauty secrets from the vineyards*. 261pp. 1981. New York: Dial/Delacourte.
   The first complete guide to wines and health.

1248   Michele, Arthur M. *You don't have to ache: a guide to orthotherapy*. 208pp. 1974. London: Pan Books.
   Exercises for backache, aching feet, headache, etc.

1249   Miles, *Mrs*. Eustace. *Health without meat*. 137pp. 1923. London: Methuen. First published in 1915.
   Based on Mr. Eustace Miles' well-known dietetic principle.

1250   Miller, Saul and Jo Anne Miller. *Food for thought: a new look at food and behaviour*. 202pp. 1979. Englewood Cliffs, New Jersey: Prentice-Hall.

1251   Mitchell, F.W.D. *A key to healthy and long life: the secret of healthy nutrition.* 191pp. 1922. London: C.W. Daniel.

1252   Moore, S.T. and M.P. Byers. *Vegetarian diet: what it is; and how to make it healthful and enjoyable.* 120pp. 1978. Santa Barbara, California: Woodbridge Press.

1253   Morgulis, Sergius. *Fasting and undernutrition: a biological and sociological study of inanition.* 407pp. 1923. New York: E.P. Dutton.

1254   Moule, Tom W. *Nature cure in a nutshell.* 63pp. 1976. Wellingborough, Northamptonshire: Thorsons. First published in 1953.

1255   Moyer, Anne (editor). *The fiber factor: how to stay healthy with bran and high fiber foods.* 146pp. 1976. Emmaus, Pennsylvania: Rodale.

1256   Moyle, Alan. *Conquering constipation: the natural guide to intestinal health.* 126pp. 1982. Wellingborough, Northamptonshire: Thorsons. First published in 1976.

1257   Moyle, A. *Diets to help acne.* 47pp. 1981. Wellingborough, Northamptonshire: Thorsons.

1258   Moyle, A. *Diets to help bronchial troubles.* 47pp. 1981. Wellingborough, Northamptonshire: Thorsons.

1259   Moyle, A. *Diets to help catarrh.* 48pp. 1980. Wellingborough, Northamptonshire: Thorsons.

1260   Moyle, A. *Diets to help constipation.* 46pp. 1980. Wellingborough, Northamptonshire: Thorsons.

1261   Moyle, A. *Insomnia: end the misery of sleepless nights.* 62pp. 1982. Wellingborough, Northamptonshire: Thorsons.

1262   Moyle, A. *Molasses and nutrition.* 64pp. 1976. Wellingborough, Northamptonshire: Thorsons.

1263   Moyle, A. *Natural healing.* 61pp. 1979. Wellingborough, Northamptonshire: Thorsons.

1264   Moyle, A. *Natural health for the elderly.* 128pp. 1975. Wellingborough, Northamptonshire: Thorsons.

1265   Moyle, A. *Nature cure explained*. 185pp. 1950. London: Health For All.

1266   Moyle, A. *Nature cure for asthma and hay fever*. 63pp. 1982. Wellingborough, Northamptonshire: Thorsons.

1267   Moyle, A. *Self-treatment for digestive troubles*. 64pp. 1982. Wellingborough, Northamptonshire: Thorsons.

1268   Munro, Daniel C. *Man alive you're half dead! A physician tells you how to eat your way to glowing health ... and stay there*. 209pp. 1950. New York: Bartholomew House.

1269   Muramato, Noboru. *Healing ourselves*. 150pp. 1973. New York: Avon Books.

1270   Murray, Frank. *Program your heart for health*. 363pp. 1977. New York: Larchmont Books.

1271   Nature Cure Educational Association. *The health and nature cure handbook: a complete authoritative and independent guide to nature cure and healthy living*. Volume 1: 166pp. 1931. Volume 2: 199pp. 1932. London: Nature Cure Educational Association.

1272   Newton-Fenbow, Peter. *A time to heal: a personal testimony of Dr. Issels' cancer treatment*. 192pp. 1971. London: Souvenir Press.

1273   Nightingale, Michael. *Diets to help headaches*. 47pp. 1981. Wellingborough, Northamptonshire: Thorsons.

1274   Nittler, Alan. *A new breed of doctor*. 202pp. 1974. New York: Pyramid Publications.
   A technical, but interesting introduction to nutrition.

1275   Norfolk, Donald. *Fit for life: a blueprint for healthy living*. 288pp. 1980. Feltham, Middlesex: Hamlyn.

1276   Norris, P.E. *About honey: nature's elixir for health and energy*. 64pp. 1983. Wellingborough, Northamptonshire: Thorsons.

1277   Norris, P.E. *About molasses: natural remedy, natural food*. 62pp. 1980. Wellingborough, Northamptonshire: Thorsons.

1278   Norris, P.E. *About yeasts: a unique and concentrated natural food.* 64pp. 1980. Wellingborough, Northamptonshire: Thorsons.

1279   Norris, P.E. *About yogurt.* 63pp. 1980. Wellingborough, Northamptonshire: Thorsons.

1280   Nugent, Nancy and the editors of *Prevention* magazine. *Food and nutrition.* 176pp. 1984. Emmaus, Pennsylvania: Rodale.
Shows how important proper nutrition is to a sense of health and well-being.

1281   Null, Gary. *Food combining handbook.* 140pp. 1976. New York: Pyramid Publications. First published in 1973.
A very good, informative book.

1282   Null, G. *The new vegetarian: building your health through natural eating.* 350pp. 1978. New York: William Morrow.
An extremely complete book on vegetarianism.

1283   Null, G. *Protein for vegetarians.* 189pp. 1975. New York: Pyramid Publications.

1284   Null, G. and Steve Null. *The complete handbook of nutrition.* 413pp. 1980. New York: Dell Books. A useful and comprehensive general book on nutrition.

1285   Null, G. and S. Null. *Handbook of skin and hair.* 176pp. 1976. New York: Pyramid Publications.

1286   Null, C. and S. Null. *Why your stomach hurts: a handbook of digestion and nutrition.* 224p. 1979. New York: Dell Books.
A detailed reference work.

1287   Nutrition Search Inc. *Nutrition almanac.* 279pp. 1979. New York: McGraw-Hill.
The best single sourcebook on nutrition. Highly recommended.

1288   Oldfield, Josiah. *The dry diet cure.* 140pp. 1933. London: C.W. Daniel. First published in 1925.

1289   Oldfield, J. *Fasting for health and life.* 186pp. 1934. London: C.W. Daniel. First published in 1924.

1290   Oliver, Martha H. *Add a few sprouts to eat better for less money.* 126pp. 1975. New Canaan, Connecticut: Keats.
  Nutritional and medicinal value of sprouts.

1291   O'Meara, E.J. *Medical guide for India, and book of prescriptions.* 695pp. 1924. London: Butterworth and Co., Medical Publishers.
  Looks at naturopathic and allopathic treatments.

1292   Ott, John N. *Health and light.* 222pp. 1981. London and Dulverton, Somerset: Watkins Publishing.
  Explores light as a nutrient.

1293   Padus, Emrika. *The woman's encyclopedia of health and natural healing.* 640pp. 1984. Emmaus, Pennsylvania: Rodale.
  Practical and comprehensive.

1294   Page, Melvin and H. Leon Abrams, Jnr. *Your body is your best doctor.* 236pp. 1974. New Canaan, Connecticut: Keats.

1295   Palmer, Margaret. *Lessons on massage.* 320pp. 1942. London: Baillière, Tindall and Cox.

1296   Passwater, Richard A. *Dr. Richard Passwater's nutrition workbook.* 1984. New Canaan, Connecticut: Keats. An authoritative guide.

1297   Pauls, Arthur Lincoln. *Shivambu Kalpa.* 145pp. 1978. Cheshunt, Hertfordshire: Ortho-Bionomy Publishing.

1298   Pearce, Ian C.B. *The holistic approach to cancer.* 95pp. 1983. Alexandria, Dunbartonshire: R. Findlay.

1299   Pelstring, Linda and Jo-Ann Hauck. *Food to improve your health.* 221pp. 1974. New York: Walker.
  A reference book.

1300   Pemble, Edna. *Self-help for your arthritis.* 71pp. 1981. London: Sheldon Press.

1301   Peppard, Harold M. *Better sight without glasses.* 162pp. 1938. New York: Eye Health, Inc.

1302   Peterson, Vicki. *Eat your way to health.* 208pp. 1982. London: Penguin.
  A comprehensive look at food and health.

1303   Peterson, V. *Natural food catalog*. 160pp. 1978. New York: Arco.

1304   Pfeiffer, Carl. *Schizophrenias, yours and mine*. 158pp. 1977. New York: Jove Publications.

1305   Phillips, David A. *Guide to nutritional factors in foods*. 128pp. 1984. Santa Barbara, California: Woodbridge Press.

1306   Phillips, D.A. *New dimensions in health: from soil to psyche*. 301pp. 1983. North Ryde, Australia: Angus and Robertson.
        A comprehensive work.

1307   Phillips, F. *Out of darkness into light. Master guide to health*. 139pp. n.d. Edinburgh: By author.
        Of historical interest.

1308   Phillips, G. *Banish ill health: the art of being well and living long. Principles and practice of nature care explained*. 74pp. 1950. Ashingdon, Essex: C. W. Daniel.

1309   Platen, M. *The new curative treatment of disease: handbook of hygienic rules of life, health culture and the cure of ailments without the aid of drugs. An invaluable household and family guide for the healthy and the ailing*. Volume 1: 741pp. n.d. Volume 2: 1579pp. n.d. London: Bong and Co.

1310   Pleshette, Janet. *Health on your plate: a complete guide to food therapy, the natural way to fight disease*. 432pp. 1983. London: Hamlyn Paperbacks.

1311   Polunin, Miriam. *The right way to eat: to feel good—or even better*. 166pp. 1984. London: J. M. Dent and Sons.
        Includes a guide to food additives and the EEC numbers.

1312   Polunin, M. *Skin troubles: practical remedial measures, including a special seven-day diet*. 96pp. 1984. Melbourne, Victoria: Science of Life Books.

1313   Polunin, M. (editor). *The health and fitness handbook: a family guide*. 256pp. 1981. Farncombe, Surrey: Here's Health (with Windward).

1313A   Popov, Ivan. *Stay young*. 286pp. 1975. New York: Grosset and Dunlap.

1314   Porter, Charles Stanford. *Milk diet as a remedy for chronic disease.* 280pp. 1919. Los Gatos, California: By author. First published in 1905.

1315   Powell, Eric F.W. *Health from earth, air and water.* 64pp. 1970. Holsworthy, Devon: Health Science Press.
Explains how the elements can be used for health and healing.

1316   Powell, E.F.W. *Health from the kitchen.* 63pp. 1973. Holsworthy, Devon: Health Science Press.
A fascinating book.

1317   Powell, E.F.W. *A home course in nutrition.* 105pp. 1978. Holsworthy, Devon: Health Science Press.
A helpful, practical guide.

1318   Powell, E.F.W. *A simple way to successful living.* 87pp. 1951. Kingswood, Surrey: The World's Work (1913) Ltd.
Simple, natural ways to health.

1319   Powell, Milton. *How to strengthen weak nerves.* 64pp. 1981. Wellingborough, Northamptonshire: Thorsons.

1320   Powell, M. *An outline of naturopathic psychotherapy.* 162pp. 1967. London: British College of Naturopathy and Osteopathy.

1321   Powell, *Mrs.* Milton. *Eating for perfect health: food reform and meatless cookery. The principles and practice of food reform simply and clearly explained, including recipes.* 174pp. 1932. London: Athletic Publications. First published in 1926.

1322   *Prevention* magazine (editors). *The natural way to a healthy skin.* 202pp. 1972. Emmaus, Pennsylvania: Rodale.
Based on articles from *Prevention* magazine.

1323   *Prevention* magazine (editors). *'Prevention's' New encyclopedia of common diseases.* 1104pp. 1984. Emmaus, Pennsylvania: Rodale.
An up-dated version of one of the health classics.

1324   Price, C.S. *The improvement of sight by natural methods: a complete treatise upon the newer method of treating all conditions of imperfect sight by natural means, and obviating the necessity for glasses, drugs or operations.* 258pp. 1948. London: Chapman and Hall.
Relaxation, imagination, exercises. etc.

1325   Price, Weston A. *Nutrition and physical degeneration. A comparison of primitive and modern diets and their effects.* 526pp. 1979. La Mesa, California: Price–Pottenger Nutrition Foundation. First published in 1939.
A landmark study of the effects of 'civilized' foods on health.

1326   Pritikin, Nathan and Patrick M. McGrady, Jnr. *The Pritikin programme for diet and exercise.* 446pp. 1979. New York: Grosset and Dunlap.

1327   Puderbach, P. *The massage operator.* 180pp. 1925. Butler, New Jersey: Benedict Lust Publications.

1328   Quick, Clifford. *Diets to help hyper-tension.* 48pp. 1980. Wellingborough, Northamptonshire: Thorsons.

1329   Quick, C. *Fact book on sinusitis, bronchitis and emphysema and their natural treatment.* 64pp. 1975. New Canaan, Connecticut: Keats.

1330   Quick, C. *Nature cure for bronchitis and emphysema.* 64pp. 1983. Wellingborough, Northamptonshire: Thorsons.

1331   Quick, C. *Nature cure for cystitis.* 64pp. 1981. Wellingborough, Northamptonshire: Thorsons.
A simply written account.

1332   Quick, C. *Nature cure for sinusitis.* 64pp. 1980. Wellingborough, Northamptonshire: Thorsons.

1333   Quick, C. *Why endure rheumatism and arthritis?* 201pp. 1982. London: Unwin.
Diets and exercises.

1334   Rabagliati, A. *Air, food and exercises: an essay on the predisposing causes of disease.* 559pp. 1904. London: Baillière, Tindall and Cox.

1335   Rama, Swami. *A practical guide to holistic health.* 133pp. 1980. Honesdale, Pennsylvania: The Himalayan International Institute.

1336   Ramacharaka, Yogi. *The practical water cure.* 123pp. 1937. Jacksonville, Florida: Yogi Publication Society.
A comprehensive survey of various water cures practised in India and the Orient.

1337   Ramsey, Vic. *Healing and the vitamin factor*. 159pp. 1983. Basingstoke: Marshalls.
   Deals with diet, exercises, stress disorders, etc.

1338   Rapp, Doris. *Allergies and the hyperactive child*. 224pp. 1979. New York: Simon and Schuster.
   A non-technical and informative book.

1339   Rapp, D. *Allergies and your family*. 352pp. 1980. New York: Sterling Publishing Company.
   An authoritative text.

1340   Ray, Matthew B. *On prescribing physical treatment*. 179pp. 1929. London: William Heinemann Medical Books.
   A textbook for practitioners, including water therapy, massage and electrical therapy.

1341   Read, Anne, Carol Ilstrup and Margaret Gammon. *Edgar Cayce on diet and health*. 191pp. 1969. New York: Warner Books.
   Includes selections from the Cayce readings.

1342   Reilly, Harold J. and Ruth Hagy Brod. *The Edgar Cayce handbook for health through drugless therapy*. 348pp. 1975. New York: Macmillan.
   One of the most comprehensive and useful books on Cayce's health ideas.

1343   Reinhardt, Charles. *120 years of life: the book of sour milk treatment*. 60pp. 1910. London: The London Publishing Company Ltd.
   What the treatment is, and what it does.

1344   Reuben, David. *The save your life diet*. 160pp. 1976. London: Michael Joseph.
   A pioneering work that remains one of the most popular books about the role of fibre in health.

1345   Robinson, F.A. *Attacking and arresting arthritis*. 100pp. 1945. Toronto, Canada: Health Book Supply Co.
   Nature cure.

1346   Rodale, J.I. *Health treasury*. 320pp. 1968. Berkhamsted, Hertfordshire: Rodale.

1347   Rodale, J.I. *Natural health, sugar and the criminal mind*. 189pp. 1968. New York: Pyramid Publications.
   The link between modern diet and behavioural problems.

1348   Rodale, J.I. *The natural way to better eyesight*. 127pp. 1968. New York: Pyramid Publications.
Sunflower seeds, vitamins, diets, Bates system, etc.

1349   Rodale, J.I. *Rodale's system for mental power and natural health*. 157pp. 1968. New York: Pyramid Publications.
Mental power and natural health.

1350   Rodale, J.I. *Winning the battle against arthritis*. 96pp. n.d. Berkhamsted, Hertfordshire: Rodale.

1351   Rodale, J.I. (editor). *The health builder*: formally called 'Volume 2 of *The health finder*.' 1024pp. 1957. Emmaus, Pennsylvania: Rodale.
Alphabetically arranged.

1352   Rodale, J.I. (editor). *The health finder: an encyclopaedia of health information from the preventive point-of-view*. 946pp. 1959. Emmaus, Pennsylvania: Rodale. First published in 1954.

1353   Rodale, J.I. and staff of *Prevention* magazine (edited by Harold J. Taub). *Natural health and pregnancy: a handbook for mothers-to-be*. 320pp. 1968. New York: Pyramid Publications.

1354   Rodale, J.I. and staff of *Prevention* magazine. *Nerves, emotions and your health*. 62pp. 1963. Emmaus, Pennsylvania: Rodale.

1355   Rodale, J.I. and staff of *Prevention* magazine (editors). *Encyclopedia for healthful living*. 1055pp. 1960. Emmaus, Pennsylvania: Rodale.

1356   Rodale, J.I. and staff of *Prevention* magazine (editors). *The health seeker*. 928pp. 1962. Emmaus, Pennsylvania: Rodale.
Reprint material on a variety of diseases and health problems.

1357   Roe, D. *Drug induced nutritional deficiencies*. 1976. Westport, Connecticut: AVI Publishing Co.

1358   Rohé, Fred. *Metabolic ecology: a way to win the cancer war*. 225pp. 1982. Winfield, Kansas: Wedgestone Press.

1359   Rosaries-Berrett, Marilyn. *Do you really need eye glasses?* 126pp. 1974. New York: Hart Publishing Company.
A good book on eyesight improvement.

1360   Rosenburg, Harold S. *Nutrition and stress: only total health awareness can help us survive.* 25pp. 1983. New Canaan, Connecticut: Keats.

1361   Ross, Shirley. *Fasting: the super diet.* 118pp. 1978. London: Pan Books.
A well researched general survey.

1362   Rossiter, Frederick. *Water health for healing.* 128pp. 1984. Santa Barbara, California: Woodbridge Press.
A practical guide.

1363   Rowen, Lilian. *No more headaches: a simple exercise programme for complete relief.* 31pp. 1982. London: Sheldon Press.

1364   Rowsell, Henry and Helen MacFarlane. *Henry' Bee herbal: modern applications of honey therapy.* 128pp. 1974. Wellingborough, Northamptonshire: Thorsons.

1365   Russell, W. Kerr. *Colonic irrigation.* 191pp. 1932. Edinburgh: E. and S. Livingstone.
The history, practice and use of colonic irrigation.

1366   Sams, Craig. *About macrobiotics: the way of eating.* 61pp. 1983. Wellingborough, Northamptonshire: Thorsons. First published in 1972.

1367   Saxon, Edgar J. *1878–1956: A sense of wonder.* 66pp. n.d. London: C.W. Daniel.
Essays on 'right living—nature's way'.

1368   Saxon, E.J. *Sensible food for all: in Britain and the temperate zones.* 133pp. 1939. London: C.W. Daniel.
Good nutrition and health.

1369   Sanders, T.A.B. and Frey R. Ellis. *Vegan nutrition.* 23pp. 1979. Leatherhead, Surrey: The Vegan Society.

1370   Sanderson-Wells, T.H. *Sun diet, or, live food for live Britons.* 100pp. 1939. London: John Bale, Sons and Curnow Ltd.
Looks at nutrition and digestion.

1371 Scharffenberg, John A. *Problems with meat: are there hidden hazards in our high meat diet?* 110pp. 1979. Santa Barbara, California: Woodbridge Press.

1372 Schauss, Alexander. *Diet, crime and delinquency.* 118pp. 1981. Berkeley, California: Parker House.

1373 Schellberg, O.B. *Colonic therapy in the treatment of disease.* 202pp. 1923. New York: Schellberg Institute.
Of historical interest.

1374 Schneider, L.L. and Robert B. Stone. *Old fashioned health remedies that work best.* 227pp. 1977. Englewood Cliffs, New Jersey: Prentice-Hall.

1375 Schroemaker, Josephine. *Gentle is the way: the Montgomery methods of massage and vitalization.* 68pp. 1981. Marina Del Rey, California: De Vorss.
A clearly written guide.

1376 Science of Life Books (editors). *The common cold.* 64pp. 1980. Melbourne, Victoria: Science of Life Books.
A discussion of causes and remedies based on natural treatments.

1377 Science of Life Books (editors). *Glands and your health.* 64pp. 1975. Melbourne, Victoria: Science of Life Books.

1378 Science of Life Books (editors). *High blood pressure.* 64pp. 1980. Melbourne, Victoria: Science of Life Books.

1379 Science of Life Books (editors). *Improve your sight without glasses: achieving better eyesight with exercise and diet.* 62pp. 1981. Melbourne, Victoria: Science of Life Books.
Outlines a new optical science.

1380 Science of Life Books (editors). *Liver ailments and common disorders: showing that a correct diet is the key to health.* 63pp. 1981. Melbourne, Victoria: Science of Life Books.

1381 Science of Life Books (editors). *Massage at your fingertips.* 62pp. 1980. Melbourne, Victoria: Science of Life Books.
General discussion of therapeutic massage.

1382 Science of Life Books (editors). *Nerve troubles: nutritional treatment of neuritis, neuralgia, neurasthenia and nervous debility.* 63pp. 1980. Melbourne, Victoria: Science of Life Books.

1383   Science of Life Books (editors). *Rheumatism and arthritis: an outline of common causes and safe corrective measures including vitamin therapy, hydrotherapy and the ideal day's diet.* 60pp. 1971. Melbourne, Victoria: Science of Life Books.

1384   Science of Life Books (editors). *Skin troubles: practical remedial measures including a special seven-day diet.* 96pp. 1984. Melbourne, Victoria: Science of Life Books.

1385   Science of Life Books (editors). *Stomach ulcers and acidity: remedies for avoiding needless pain and suffering.* 63pp. 1983. Melbourne, Victoria: Science of Life Books.

1386   Scott, Cyril. *Cider vinegar. Nature's great health-promoter and safest cure of obesity.* 40pp. n.d. London: Athene.

1387   Scott, C. *Sleeplessness: prevention and cure by natural methods.* 46pp. 1980. Wellingborough, Northamptonshire: Thorsons.

1388   Scrutton, Robert J. *Eating right is beautiful.* 176pp. 1984. Sudbury, Suffolk: Neville Spearman.

1389   Scrutton, R.J. *Nature's way to nutrition and vibrant health.* 173pp. 1977. Hollywood, California: Wilshire Book Company.

1390   Senate Select Committee on Nutrition and Human Needs. *Dietary goals for the United States.* 178pp. 1980. Berkeley, California: Parker House.
    An explanation of the dietary goals, reasons for dietary change, and additional information about the food habits of Americans. The original report was made in 1977; this is an updated version.

1391   Shackleton, B. *The grape cure.* 128pp. 1983. Wellingborough, Northamptonshire: Thorsons.

1392   Shears, C. Curtis. *Nutritional science and health education.* 140pp. 1978. Gloucester: The Nutritional Science Research Institute.
    A carefully researched and documented book for the expert.

1393   Shears, Elizabeth. *Why do we eat?* 138pp. 1979. Gloucester: The Nutritional Science Research institute.
    A practical and unique book.

1394   Sheinkin, D., M. Schacter and R. Hutton. *Food, mood and mind.* 304pp. 1979. New York: Warner Books.
Probably one of the best books on food and ecological allergies.

1395   Shelton, Herbert M. *The basic principles of natural hygiene.* 660pp. 1944. San Antonio, Texas: Dr. Shelton's Health School.

1396   Shelton, H.M. *Fasting can save your life.* 195pp. 1981. Bridgeport, Connecticut: Natural Hygiene Press. First published in 1964.
Reviews the whole area of fasting.

1397   Shelton, H.M. *Fasting for renewal of life.* 314pp. 1978. Bridgeport, Connecticut: Natural Hygiene Press.
One of the most comprehensive and scholarly treatments of the subject.

1398   Shelton, H.M. *Food combining made easy.* 63pp. 1982. San Antonio, Texas: Willow Publishing Inc. First published in 1951.
Summarizes Shelton's views.

1399   Shelton, H.M. *Health for the millions.* 314pp. 1968. Bridgeport, Connecticut: Natural Hygiene Press.
A good introduction to the natural hygiene story.

1400   Shelton, H.M. *The hygienic care of children.* 473pp. 1970. Bridgeport, Connecticut: Natural Hygiene Press.
One of the only books of its kind.

1401   Shelton, H.M. *The hygienic system.* 7 volumes. 1969. Mokelumne Hill, California: Health Research. First published in 1937.

1402   Shelton, H.M. *An introduction to natural hygiene.* 92pp. 1963. Moklumne Hill, California: Health Research. First published in 1922.

1403   Shelton, H.M. *The joys of getting well.* 112pp. 1957. San Antonio, California: Dr. Shelton's Health School.

1404   Shelton, H.M. *The road to health via natural hygiene.* 69pp. 1958. New York: The Health Guild.

1405   Shelton, H.M. *The science and fine art of fasting.* 384pp. 1978. Bridgeport, Connecticut: Natural Hygiene Press. First published in 1934.
Recommended.

1406   Shelton, H.M. *Superior nutrition.* 197pp. 1978. San Antonio, Texas: Dr. Shelton's Health School.
A comprehensive text on Shelton's philosophy of diet.

1407   Simons, P. *Nutrition: everything you need to know to ensure healthy wholesome eating.* 91p. 1978. Wellingborough, Northamptonshire: Thorsons.
A brief, clear survey of the fundamentals of nutrition.

1408   Simpkins, R. Brooks. *New light on the eyes: revolutionary and scientific discoveries which indicate extensive reform and radical improvement in the treatment of diseases such as cataract and glaucoma.* 142pp. 1958. London: Vincent Stuart Ltd.

1409   Simpkins, R.B. *Visible ray therapy of the eyes.* 100pp. 1963. Rustington, Sussex: Health Science Press.
For cataracts, glaucoma, retinitis, etc. A natural medicine for the eyes.

1410   Singer, Francis G. *Physiolelsis: a philosophy productive of a high standard of health, fitness and physical efficiency by clearly planned and consciously directed effort.* 87pp. 1937. Brisbane, Australia: John Mills Himself, Printer and Publisher. This first edition was for private circulation only.
Looks at food, health and disease.

1411   Sneddon, J. Russell. *Food way to health.* 163pp. 1946. Glasgow: Wm. Maclellan.

1412   Sneddon, J.R. *Healing yourself with water.* 64pp. 1977. Wellingborough, Northamptonshire: Thorsons.

1413   Sneddon, J.R. *High blood pressure.* 64pp. 1983. Wellingborough, Northamptonshire: Thorsons.

1414   Sneddon, J.R. *How to cure catarrhal deafness.* 64pp. 1981. Wellingborough, Northamptonshire: Thorsons.

1415   Sneddon, J.R. *Natural hair care.* 64pp. 1981. Wellingborough, Northamptonshire: Thorsons.

1416   Sneddon, J.R. *The natural treatment of liver troubles.* 63pp. 1980. Wellingborough, Northamptonshire: Thorsons.

1417   Sneddon, J.R. *The nature cure treatment of gastric and duodenal ulceration.* 64pp. 1982. Wellingborough, Northamptonshire: Thorsons.

1418   Sneddon, J.R. *The nature cure for rheumatic ailments.* 63pp. 1980. Wellingborough, Northamptonshire: Thorsons.

1419   Sneddon, J.R. *The nature cure treatment for varicose veins and ulcers.* 63pp. 1982. Wellingborough, Northamptonshire: Thorsons.

1420   Sneddon, J.R. *The successful treatment of catarrh.* 60pp. 1980. Wellingborough, Northamptonshire: Thorsons.

1421   Sneddon, J.R. *The successful treatment of hair disorders.* 64pp. 1974. Wellingborough, Northamptonshire: Thorsons.

1422   Speight, Phyllis. *Overcoming rheumatism and arthritis.* 64pp. 1974. Wellingborough, Northamptonshire: Thorsons.
        Includes naturopathy as well as herbs and homoeopathy.

1423   Stanway, Andrew. *Taking the rough with the smooth: dietary fiber and your health. The essential handbook.* 281pp. 1981. London: Pan Books.
        One of the most reasoned, authoritative books on the subject.

1424   Stuart, Elma. *What must I do to get well? And how can I keep so?* 314pp. 1895. Wokingham, Berkshire: By author.
        Based on the Salisbury treatment, which looks at health and nutrition.

1425   Subak-Sharpe, Genell. *The natural high fiber life saving diet.* 190pp. 1976. New York: Grosset and Dunlap.
        Reviews the medical research.

1426   Suren, Hans. *Man and sunlight.* 196pp. 1927. Slough: The Solux Publishing Co
        Looks at the effect of sunlight on health.

1427   Sussman, V. *The vegetarian alternative.* 286pp. 1978. Emmaus, Pennsylvania: Rodale.
        A well researched guide.

1428   Swank, Ray L. *The multiple sclerosis diet book: a low-fat diet for the treatment of multiple sclerosis, heart disease and stroke.* 326pp. 1977. Garden City, New York: Doubleday.

1429   Szekely, Edmond Bordeaux (translator). *The Essene gospel of peace.* 72pp. 1975. San Diego, California: Academy Books.
   A translation of a third-century Aramaic manuscript, which gives Christ's views on healing and health.

1430   Szekely, E.B. (translated by L. Purcell Weaver). *Medicine to-morrow. An introduction to cosmotherapy.* 289pp. 1938. London: C.W. Daniel.

1431   Szekely, E.B. *Therapeutic fasting.* 28pp. 1938. London: C.W. Daniel.

1432   Szekely, E.B. *Three by Szekely (Book of vitamins; Book of minerals; Book of herbs).* 128pp. 1983. New Canaan, Connecticut: Keats.

1433   Tappan, F. *Healing massage techniques: a study of Eastern and Western methods.* 260pp. 1980. Reston, Virginia: Reston Publishing Company.
   Based on thirty-two years of research into all known massage techniques.

1434   Taub, Harold. *Keeping healthy in a polluted world.* 246pp. 1974. New York: Viking Penguin Inc.

1435   Terry, Robert J. *How to get well and keep well.* 204pp. n.d. London: Whitcombe and Tombs.
   Nutrition for the family. Aimed at the housewives of the day.

1436   Thompson, J. Douglas. *Eating your way to health library.* Volume 1: 254pp. 1935. Volume 2: 254pp. 1935. Volume 3: 254pp. 1935. Volume 4: 254pp. 1934. Oakland, California: Thompson Health Publications.

1437   Thompson, William R. *Living with angina.* 64pp. 1983. Wellingborough, Northamptonshire: Thorsons.

1438   Thomson, C. Leslie. *The healthy human gut: an epitomical version of J.C. Thomson's 'Constipation and our civilization'.* 40pp. 1978. Edinburgh: Kingston Clinic.

1439   Thomson, C.L. *Your sight: cure and improvement by natural means.* 99pp. 1966. London: Thorsons.

1440   Thomson, James C. *The heart: the prevention and cure of cardiac conditions.* 143pp. n.d. London: Thorsons.

1441   Thomson, J.C. *An introduction to nature cure.* 136pp. 1924. London: C.W. Daniel.

1442   Thomson, J.C. *Towards high level health.* 62pp. 1960. Edinburgh: Kingston Clinic.

1443   Thomson, J.C. *Your heart.* 78pp. 1974. London: C.W. Daniel. An informative and helpful book for heart patients.

1444   Thomson, J.C. and C. Leslie Thomson. *Healthy hair: care and restoration by natural methods.* 94pp. 1983. Wellingborough, Northamptonshire: Thorsons.

1445   Thomson, Robert. *Natural medicine.* 329pp. 1981. London: Wildwood House. A general book on naturopathy.

1446   Thurston, Emory. *Parents guide to better nutrition for tots to teens (and others).* 162pp. 1979. New Canaan, Connecticut: Keats.

1447   Tibbs, Hardwin. *The future of light.* 103pp. 1981. Dulverton, Somerset: Watkins Publishing. Discusses the relationship between health and light.

1448   Tilden, J.H. *Food: its influence as a factor in disease and health.* 250pp. 1976. New Canaan, Connecticut: Keats. One of Tilden's most important works.

1449   Tilden, J.H. *Impaired health: its cause and cure.* 2 volumes. 1960. Mokelumne Hill, California: Health Research.

1450   Tilden, J.H. *Toxemia explained.* 144pp. 1981. New Canaan, Connecticut: Keats. Originally published in 1926. A valuable work.

1451   Tobe, John H. *How to prevent and gain remission from cancer.* 353pp. 1975. St. Catherines, Ontario: Provoker Press.

1452   Turner, E.S. *Taking the cure.* 284pp. 1967. London: Michael Joseph.

1453   Turner, Roger Newman. *Diets to help control cholesterol.* 48pp. 1980. Wellingborough, Northamptonshire: Thorsons.

1454   Turner, R.N. *Diets to help hay fever and asthma.* 47pp. 1983. Wellingborough, Northamptonshire: Thorsons.

1455   Turner, R.N. *Diets to help heart disorders.* 48pp. 1980. Wellingborough, Northamptonshire: Thorsons.

1456   Turner, R.N. *First aid nature's way.* 93pp. 1978. Wellingborough, Northamptonshire: Thorsons.
Safe and effective treatments for minor ailments and injuries.

1457   Turner, R.N. *Naturopathic first aid.* 93pp. 1969. Wellingborough, Northamptonshire: Thorsons.

1458   Turner, R.N. *Naturopathic medicine: treating the person as a whole.* 155pp. 1984. Wellingborough, Northamptonshire: Thorsons.
Outlines the thinking behind naturopathy and describes the various treatments used.

1459   Turner, R.N. *Self-help for gall-bladder troubles.* 64pp. 1981. Wellingborough, Northamptonshire: Thorsons.

1460   Ulrich, Rolf (translated by Janet Ellengham). *Coffee and caffeine.* 52pp. 1958. Bristol, Avon: John Wright.

1461   Valnet, Jean. *Heal yourself with vegetables, fruit and grains.* 224pp. 1975. New York: Simon and Schuster.
A very informative encyclopaedia.

1462   Vaughan, F.W. *The new bedrock of health: an antitoxemic nature cure based on the Ebbard method of treating diseases and chronic disorders without drugs or operations.* 263pp. 1906. London: L.N. Fowler.

1463   Verrett, Jacqueline and Jean Carper. *Eating may be hazardous to your health.* 256pp. 1974. Garden City, New York: Doubleday.

1464   Vogel, A. *Swiss nature doctor: an encyclopaedic collection of helpful hints gathered from Swiss folklore of healing.* 512pp. 1980. Teufen, Switzerland: A. Vogel Verlag.

1465 Vosnjak, Mitja. *Miracle of propolils.* 96pp. 1980. Wellingborough, Northamptonshire: Thorsons.
The story of the Yugoslavian rediscovery of the efficacy of propolis.

1466 Wade, Carlson. *All natural pain relievers.* 227pp. 1975. Englewood Cliffs, New Jersey: Prentice-Hall.
A good reference book.

1467 Wade, C. *Bee pollen and your health.* 117pp. 1978. New Canaan, Connecticut: Keats.
A comprehensive account.

1468 Wade, C. *Emotional health and nutrition.* 155pp. 1971. Bergenfield, New Jersey: Award Sales.

1469 Wade, C. *Fact book on arthritis, nutrition and natural therapy.* 124pp. 1976. New Canaan, Connecticut: Keats.

1470 Wade, C. *Fact book on fats, oils and cholesterol.* 125pp. 1973. New Canaan, Connecticut: Keats.
A useful reference book.

1471 Wade, C. *Helping your health with enzymes.* 224pp. 1981. New York: Arco. First published in 1966.

1472 Wade, C. *Hyper-tension (high blood pressure) and your diet.* 158pp. 1975. New Canaan, Connecticut: Keats.
A useful compendium of information.

1473 Wade, C. *Instant health: the nature way.* 220pp. n.d. London: Tandem Books.

1474 Wade, C. *What's in it for you.* 170pp. 1981. New Canaan, Connecticut: Keats.
Looks at over four hundred health foods, vitamins, supplements, etc.

1475 Waerland, Are. *The cauldron of disease.* 298pp. 1934. London: David Nutt (A. G. Berry).
Instructs the reader in health and happiness.

1476 Waerland, A. *Health is your birthright.* 88pp. n.d. Bern, Switzerland: Humata Publishing.
Describes the Waerland system and its underlying philosophy.

1477   Waerland, Ebba. *Cancer: a disease of civilisation.* 54pp. 1976. St. Catherines, Ontario: Provoker Press.

1478   Waerland, Ebba. *Rebuilding health: the Waerland method of natural therapy.* 252pp. 1966. London: James Clarke.
A detailed account of the Waerland system.

1479   Wale, J.O. (editor). *Tidy's massage and remedial exercises.* 510pp. 1978. Bristol, Avon: John Wright.

1480   Walker, Caroline and Geoffrey Cannon. *The food scandal.* 190pp. 1984. London: Century.
Explains in lay terms the implications of the report of the National Advisory Committee on Nutrition.

1481   Walker, N.W. *Become younger.* 204pp. 1949. Phoenix, Arizona: Norwalk Press.
This is the author's most complete philosophical work.

1482   Walker, N.W. *Fresh vegetable and fruit juices.* 161pp. 1983. Phoenix, Arizona: O'Sullivan, Woodside and Company.
A comprehensive discussion of the nutritional and healing properties of many juices.

1483   Walker, N.W. *The natural way to vibrant health.* 140ppp. 1983. Phoenix, Arizona: O'Sullivan, Woodside and Company.

1484   Walker, N.W. *Raw vegetable juices.* 175pp. 1982. New York: Jove Publications. First published in 1936.
A classic work.

1485   Walker, N.W. *Water can undermine your health.* 102pp. 1974. Phoenix, Arizona: O'Sullivan, Woodside and Company.

1486   Warmbrand, Max. *The encyclopedia of health and nutrition.* 468pp. 1964. London: Souvenir Press.
A valuable work.

1487   Warmbrand, M. *Living without pain.* 157pp. 1966. New York: Groton Press.

1488   Warmbrand, M. *New hope for arthritis sufferers.* 153pp. 1968. Wellingborough, Northamptonshire: Thorsons.

1489   Warmbrand, M. *Overcoming arthritis and other rheumatic diseases*. 220pp. 1976. Old Greenwich, Connecticut: Devin-Adair.
A practical and simple book.

1490   Webb-Johnson, Cecil. *Diet and disease*. 157pp. 1928. London: Selwyn and Blount.

1491   Weller, Charles and Brian Richard Boylan. *How to live with hypoglycemia*. 160pp. 1982. New York: Jove Publications.
A thorough guide.

1492   Welsh, Philip. *How to be free from arthritis*. 107pp. 1974. Santa Barbara, California: Woodbridge Press.

1493   Wendel, Paul. *Bloodless surgery: naturopathic technic and treatment*. 86pp. n.d. Wentzville, Missouri: W.G. Bazan.

1494   Wendel, P. *Standardized naturopathy: the science and art of natural healing*. 154pp. 1951. Brooklyn, New York: By author.

1495   Wertheim, Alfred. *Natural poisons in natural foods*. 210pp. 1974. Secaucus, New Jersey: Lyle Stuart.
A well researched review.

1496   Wesley, John. *Primitive remedies*. 144pp. 1984. Santa Barbara, California: Woodbridge Press.
The most popular work of John Wesley, the great Methodist reformer.

1497   West, Oudia. *The magic of massage: a new and holistic approach*. 192pp. 1984. London: Century.
Describes many techniques useful for treating a number of complaints.

1498   Wheatley, Michael. *A way of living: how to achieve natural health*. 378pp. 1982. London: Unwin. First published in 1977.

1499   White, George Starr. *The natural way, or, my work*. 954pp. 1924. Name of publisher not given.
A wonderfully eccentric book.

1500   White, G.S., Arthur Voss, J.H. Tilden, Chris Gian-Cursio, Hebert Shelton and Jethro Kloss. *Asthma, catarrh, hayfever and sinusitis*. 53pp. n.d. Mokelumne Hill, California: Health Research.
Reprints from rare, out-of-print books on natural healing.

1501   White, Julius Gilbert. *Abundant health, expanding the learn how to be well system of living.* 437pp. 1944. Privately published by author.

1502   Whitehead, Stanley B. *Everyday fare for fitness.* 166pp. 1939. London: John Lane, The Bodley Head.

1503   Whitehouse, Geoffrey T. *Everywoman's guide to natural health.* 159pp. 1981. Wellingborough, Northamptonshire: Thorsons.

1504   Whitehouse, G.T. *Why health foods?* 95pp. 1968. Farncombe, Surrey: Here's Health.

1505   Wigmore, Ann. *Why suffer?* 219pp. 1964. Boston, Massachusetts: Hippocrates Health Institute.
A personal account of the uses of wheatgerm.

1506   Wigmore, A. *You are your own healer.* 207pp. 1979. Boston, Massachusetts: Hippocrates Health Institute.

1507   Wilkinson, Marcia. *Migraine and headaches.* 108pp. 1982. London: Martin Dunitz.

1508   Williams, Roger J. *Biochemical individuality: the basis for the genetotrophic concept.* 214pp. 1979. New York: John Wiley and Sons.

1509   Williams, R.J. *Nutrition in a nutshell.* 171pp. 1962. Garden City, New York: Doubleday.
A book for the lay person who wants to know more about nutrition.

1510   Williams, R.J. *Prevention of alcoholism through nutrition.* 160pp. 1981. New York: Bantam Books.
An important work.

1511   Williams, R.J. *The wonderful world within you: your inner nutritional environment.* 1977. New York: Bantam Books.

1512   Wilson, Frank. *Food for the golden age.* 250pp. 1954. Ashingdon, Rochford, Essex: C.W. Daniel.

1513   Wilson, F. *Kelp.* 95pp. 1979. Wellingborough, Northamptonshire: Thorsons.

1514   Wilson, Jas. W. *The new hygiene: a drugless remedy for all diseases, health, longevity.* 315pp. 1910. London: G.P. Putman's Sons, Publishers.

1515   Wood, Elizabeth. *Beard's massage: principles and techniques.* 185pp. 1974. London: W.B. Saunders.

1516   Woody, Robert Henley. *The use of massage in facilitating holistic health.* 125pp. 1980. Springfield, Illinois: Charles C. Thomas.
Based on multidisciplinary research, this book will be useful to a variety of health professionals.

1517   Wrench, G.T. *The wheel of health: the sources of long life and health among the Hunza.* 146pp. 1972. New York: Schocken Books.

1518   Wright, Hannal. *Swallow it whole: the New Statesman's survival guide to the food industry.* 63pp. 1981. London: New Statesman.

1519   Wright, Jonathan V. *Dr. Wright's book of nutritional therapy: real life lessons in medicine without drugs.* 342pp. 1979. Emmaus, Pennsylvania: Rodale.
Case histories followed by a health improvement programme.

1520   Wunderlich, Ray. *Nourishing your child: a bioecologic approach.* 1984. New Canaan, Connecticut: Keats.

1521   Wunderlich, R. *Sugar and your health.* 507pp. 1982. St. Petersburg, Florida: Good Health Publications.

1522   Wynne-Tyson, Jon. *Food for a future: the ecological priority of a humane diet.* 183pp. 1975. London: Davis-Poynter.

1523   Yaller, Robert and Raye Yaller. *The health spas.* 160pp. 1984. Santa Barbara, California: Woodbridge Press.
Describes different kinds of spas, and the basic rationale of the nature cure approach.

1524   Yudkin, John. *Pure, white and deadly.* 1972. London: Davis-Poynter.

1525   Yudkin, J. *Sweet and dangerous.* 209pp. 1972. New York: Bantam Books.
Reports the findings of Yudkin's research on the connection between sugar and many diseases and degenerative conditions.

Clinical Nutrition

1526 Adams, Ruth. *The complete home guide to vitamins*. 432pp. 1976. New York: Larchmont Books.
  Includes disease prevention and treatment.

1527 Adams, R. and Frank Murray. *Body, mind and the B vitamins*. 317pp. 1983. New York: Larchmont Books.
  A clearly written account. Includes research findings.

1528 Adams, R. and F. Murray. *Improving your health with calcium and phosphorus*. 121pp. 1978. New York: Larchmont Books.

1529 Adams, R. and F. Murray. *Improving your health with vitamin A*. 125pp. 1978. New York: Larchmont Books.

1530 Adams, R. and F. Murray. *Improving your health with vitamin E*. 170pp. 1978. New York: Larchmont Books.

1531 Adams, R. and F. Murray. *Improving your health with zinc*. 122pp. 1981. New York: Larchmont Books.

1532 Adams, R. and F. Murray. *Megavitamin therapy*. 227pp. 1975. New York: Warner Books.

1533 Adams, R. and F. Murray. *Minerals: kill or cure*. 366pp. 1978. New York: Larchmont Books.
  A detailed account.

1534 Adams, R. and F. Murray. *Vitamin B$_{12}$ and folic acid*. 175pp. 1981. New York: Larchmont Books.

1535 Adams, R. and F. Murray. *The vitamin B$_6$ book*. 176pp. 1980. New York: Larchmont Books.

1536 Adams, R. and F. Murray. *Vitamin C: the powerhouse vitamin, conquers more than just colds*. 191pp. 1972. New York: Larchmont Books.

1537 Atkins, Robert C. *Dr. Atkins' nutrition breakthrough: how to treat your medical condition without drugs*. 377pp. 1981. West Caldwell, New Jersey: William Morrow.
One of the best books on nutrition.

1538 Bailey, Herbert. *Vitamin E. Your key to a healthy heart*. 203pp. 1969. New York: ARC Books.

1539 Bailey, H. *The vitamin pioneers*. 239pp. 1970. New York: Pyramid Publications.
A fascinating account.

1540 Barnes, Broda O. and Charlotte W. Barnes. *Solved: the riddle of heart attacks*. 84pp. 1977. Fort Collins, Colorado: Robinson Press.

1541 Barton-Wright, E.C. *Arthritis: cause and control. (The pantothenic acid theory)*. 40pp. n.d. London: Bunterbird.

1542 Binding, G.J. *Vegetables and herbs with a difference*. 64pp. 1977. Holsworthy, Devon: Health Science Press.
Looks at vegetables' and herbs' vitamin and mineral content.

1543 Birch, G.G. and K. Parker (editors). *Vitamin C: recent aspects of its physiological and technological importance*. 259pp. 1974. London: Applied Science Publishers.

1544 Bland, Jeffrey. Volume 1: *Choline, lecithin, inositol and other 'accessory' nutrients*. 19pp. 1982. New Canaan, Connecticut: Keats.

1545 Bland, J. *Hair tissue mineral analysis: an emergent diagnostic technique*. 80pp. 1983. Wellingborough, Northamptonshire: Thorsons.
An introduction for practitioners.

1546 Bland, J. *Nutraerobics*. 369pp. 1983. San Francisco, California: Harper and Row.
A guide to individual nutritional requirements.

1547 Bland, J. Volume 2: *Octaosanol, carnitine and other 'accessory' nutrients*. 22pp. 1982. New Canaan, Connecticut: Keats.

1548   Bland, J. (editor). *The first yearbook of clinical nutrition.* 1984. New Canaan, Connecticut: Keats.

1549   Bland, J. (editor). *Medical applications of clinical nutrition.* 321pp. 1983. New Canaan, Connecticut: Keats.

1550   Bock, Raymond. *Vitamin E: key to youthful longevity.* 62pp. 1977. New York: Arco.

1551   Bradford, Robert W. *Now that you have cancer: the laetrile metabolic program, 'orientation handbook'.* 113pp. 1979. Los Altos, California: Choice Publications.

1552   Brekhman, Izrial I. and I.F. Nesterenko. *Brown sugar and health.* 96pp. 1983. Oxford: Pergamon Press.

1553   Brekhman, I. *Man and biologically active substances: the effect of drugs, diet and pollution on health.* 89pp. 1980. Oxford: Pergamon Press.

1554   Burkitt, D. *Don't forget the fibre in your diet.* 128pp. 1983. London: Martin Dunitz.
        One of the pioneering books.

1555   Chaitow, Leon. *About laetrile: vitamin B_{17} and the fight against cancer.* 62pp. 1981. Wellingborough, Northamptonshire: Thorsons.

1556   Chaitow, L. *An end to cancer? The nutritional approach to its prevention and control.* 160pp. 1983. Wellingborough, Northamptonshire: Thorsons.
        A guide to the alternative approaches to cancer therapy based on dietary reforms and the use of laetrile.

1557   Challem, Jack Joseph. *Vitamin C updated: the great vitamin that provides optimum health and immunity.* 26pp. 1983. New Canaan, Connecticut: Keats.

1558   Cheraskin, E., W. Marshall Ringsdorf Jnr. and E. Sisley. *The vitamin C connection: getting well and staying well with vitamin C.* 299pp. 1983. Wellingborough, Northamptonshire: Thorsons.
        A scientific approach to the subject.

1559   Cleave, T.L. *The saccharine disease.* 200pp. 1974. Bristol, Avon: John Wright.
        Informative, technical and balanced.

1560   Colgan, M. *Your personal vitamin profile*. 300pp. 1983. London: Blond and Briggs.
A well researched, authoritative handbook.

1561   Consumer Guide. *The vitamin book*. 285pp. 1979. New York: Simon and Schuster.

1562   Cott, A. *Orthomolecular approach to learning difficulties*. 76pp. 1977. Novato, California: Academic Therapy Publications.

1563   Croft, J.E. *Natural relief from arthritis: a safe and effective treatment from the ocean*. 128pp. 1980. Wellingborough, Northamptonshire: Thorsons.
Nutrition therapy devised and researched by Croft.

1564   Culbert, Michael. *Freedom from cancer*. 238pp. 1976. Seal Beach, California: 76 Press.
A comprehensive review of the laetrile story.

1565   Cyan, Erwin Di. *Vitamin E and aging*. 176pp. 1972. New York: Pyramid Publications.
Includes material from the International Conference on Vitamin E and its role in cellular metabolism, held in 1971.

1566   Cyan, E.D. *Vitamins in your life*. 223pp. 1974. New York: Simon and Schuster.
An excellent survey.

1567   Dickley, Lawrence. *Clinical ecology*. 1976. Springfield, Illinois: Charles C. Thomas.

1568   Eagle, Robert. *Eating and allergy*. 209pp. 1981. Garden City, New York: Doubleday.
A thorough study of clinical ecology.

1569   Ebon, Martin. *Which vitamins do you need?* 287pp. 1981. London: Bantam Books.

1570   Eden, Jack. *The best of nature's health foods: the richest sources of natural nutrition*. 96pp. 1979. Wellingborough, Northamptonshire: Thorsons.
Looks at essential food supplements.

1571   Faelton, Sharon. *The complete book of minerals for health*. 534pp. 1981. Emmaus, Pennsylvania: Rodale.
An excellent reference book.

1572   Fisher, Leslie H. *Mineral compounds and human disease*. 129pp. 1978. Sidney, Australia: Blackmores Books.
Diagnosing for mineral deficiency.

1573   Forman, Brenda. *B₁₅: 'the miracle vitamin'*. 158pp. 1979. New York: Grosset and Dunlap.

1574   Forman, Robert. *How to control your allergies*. 256pp. 1983. New York: Larchmont Books.
Describes the clinical ecological approach.

1575   Fredericks, Carlton. *Psycho-nutrition: the diet, vitamin, and mineral way to emotional health*. 224pp. 1976. New York: Putnam Publishing Group.
Looks at megavitamin and orthomolecular therapy. Recommended.

1576   Friedman, Meyer and Ray H. Rosenman. *Type A behaviour and your heart: a radical reassessment of the causes of coronary heart disease and how to avoid it*. 266pp. 1974. London: Wildwood House.

1577   Fryer, Lee and Annette Dickinson. *Dictionary of food supplements*. 119pp. 1975. New York: Mason Charter.

1578   Garrison, Robert and Federick Hannon. *The nutrition desk reference manual*. 1984. New Canaan, Connecticut: Keats.
Information on vitamins, minerals, trace elements, etc.

1579   Gerras, Charles (editor). *The complete book of vitamins*. 814pp. 1977. Emmaus, Pennsylvania: Rodale.
An instructive overview.

1580   Gilroy, A. *Vitamins and your health*. 132pp. 1982. London: Unwin.
A readable and comprehensive reference book.

1581   Goodhart, S. Robert and Maurice Shils (editors). *Modern nutrition in health and disease*. 1153pp. 1973. Philadelphia, Pennsylvania: Lea and Febiger.
An excellent textbook of clinical nutrition.

1582   Graham, Judy. *Evening primrose oil.* 96pp. 1984. Wellingborough, Northamptonshire: Thorsons.
The full story of this natural product.

1583   Griffin, G. Edward. *World without cancer: the story of vitamin B₁₇.* 526pp. 1980. Westlake Village, California: American Media.

1584   Guenther, Ruth. *A nutritional guide for the problem drinker: the latest research on the effects of proper diet and vitamin/mineral supplementation in remedying alcohol abuse.* 24pp. 1983. New Canaan, Connecticut: Keats.

1585   Hanssen, Maurice. *E for additives.* 224pp. 1984. Wellingborough, Northamptonshire: Thorsons.
A guide to E numbers (EEC codes indicating food additives).

1586   Hanssen, M. *Spirulina: nature's diet supplement rediscovered.* 64pp. 1982. Wellingborough, Northamptonshire: Thorsons.
Describes the research to date.

1587   Hawkins, D.R. and Linus C. Pauling. *Orthomolecular psychiatry: treatment of schizophrenia.* 1973. San Francisco, California: W.H. Freeman.

1588   Hill, R. *Propolis: the natural antibiotic.* 63pp. 1981. Wellingborough, Northamptonshire: Thorsons.
A thorough overview including current research findings.

1589   Hills, Amelia Nathan. *Against the unsuspected enemy.* 181pp. 1980. Bognor Regis, Sussex: New Horizon.
A personal account of allergy-caused illness and how to overcome it with clinical ecology.

1590   Hoffer, Abram. *Vitamin B₃ (niacin): its therapeutic uses for one of the most important of the known vitamins.* 26pp. 1982. New Canaan, Connecticut: Keats.

1591   Hoffer, A. and Humphry Osmond. *How to live schizophrenia.* 224pp. 1974. Secaucus, New Jersey: Citadel Press.
A classic work.

1592   Hoffer, A. and M. Walker. *Orthomolecular nutrition.* 209pp. 1978. New Canaan, Connecticut: Keats.
An introduction to the subject.

144

1593   Hoffer, A. and others. *Megavitamin therapy in orthomolecular psychiatry*. 30pp. 1972. Cleveland, Ohio: Karpat Publishing Co.

1594   Holford, Patrick. *The whole health guide to elemental health: the book about minerals, hair mineral analysis and your health*. 208pp. 1983. Wellingborough, Northamptonshire: Thorsons.

1595   Hunter, Carol. *Vitamins: what they are and why we need them*. 96pp. 1983. Wellingborough, Northamptonshire: Thorsons.

1596   Jacobson, Michael. *How sodium nitrate can affect your health*. 55pp. 1977. Washington, DC.: Center for Science in the Public Interest.
   A well documented discussion.

1597   Kellogg, John Harvey. *The new dietetics: a guide to scientific feeding in health and disease*. 1021pp. 1923. Battle Creek, Michigan: The Modern Medicine Publiishing Co.

1598   Kittler, Glenn D. *Laetrile: nutritional control for cancer with vitamin B_{17}*. 325pp. 1978. Denver, Colorado: Nutri-Books.
   A serious study with practical guidelines.

1599   Krebs, Ernest *et al*. *The laetriles: nitrilosides in prevention and control of cancer*. 88pp. n.d. San Ysidro, California: McNaughton Foundation.
   Technical papers on laetrile treatment.

1600   Kroeger, Hanna. *Instant vitamin/mineral locator*. 70pp. 1972. Privately published by author.
   Lists vitamins and minerals.

1601   Kunin, Richard A. *Meganutrition*. 312pp. 1982. New York: McGraw-Hill.
   Primarily for the professional but accessible to the layman.

1602   Lee, William H. *Kelp, dulse and other sea supplements: nutritional treasures the ocean provides*. 23pp. 1983. New Canaan, Connecticut: Keats.

1603   Lesser, Michael. *Nutrition and vitamin therapy*. 239pp. 1981. New York: Bantam Books.
   A comprehensive guide.

1604   Lewis, Alan. *The Japanese oyster: amazing healing properties from the sea.* 62pp. 1981. Wellingborough, Northamptonshire: Thorsons.

1605   Lewis, A. *Selenium: the essential trace element you might not be getting enough of.* 96pp. 1983. Wellingborough, Northamptonshire: Thorsons.
Includes important new material on research developments.

1606   Lilliston, Lynn. *Megavitamins.* 224pp. 1975. Greenwich, Connecticut: Fawcett Publishing.
An excellent summary of the whole field.

1607   Lloyd, Eileen (editor). *Vitamin E.* 46pp. 1982. Aylesbury, Buckinghamshire: Rodale.

1608   Lloyd, E. (editor). *Vitamins.* 48pp. 1982. Aylesbury, Buckinghamshire: Rodale.

1609   McCarrison, *Sir* Robert. *Nutrition and health.* 127pp. 1982. London: The McCarrison Society.
Originally given as a lecture to the Royal Society of Arts in 1936. Also includes two earlier essays.

1610   MacFarlane, Helen B. *Arthritis: help in your own hands.* 92pp. 1982. Wellingborough, Northamptonshire: Thorsons.
Therapy based on vitamins and exercise.

1611   MacKarness, R. *Not all in the mind: how unsuspected food allergy can affect your body and your mind.* 158pp. 1976. London: Pan Books.

1612   Manner, Harold W. *The death of cancer: the story of the research involving laetrile that dropped a bombshell on orthodoxy.* 191pp. 1982. Chicago, Illinois: Advanced Century Publishing Corporation.

1613   Mervyn, Leonard. *The B vitamins: their major role in maintaining your health.* 95pp. 1983. Wellingborough, Northamptonshire: Thorsons.
A clear discussion.

1614   Mervyn, L. *The dictionary of vitamins: the complete guide to vitamins and vitamin therapy.* 224pp. 1984. Wellingborough, Northamptonshire: Thorsons.
An invaluable reference book.

1615   Mervyn, L. *Minerals and your health.* 129pp. 1981. London: Unwin.
Written for anyone concerned with nutrition and the effects of modern food processing.

1616   Mervyn, L. *Vitamin C: enemy of the common cold.* 84pp. 1982. Wellingborough, Northamptonshire: Thorsons.
A thorough discussion of recent research findings.

1617   Mervyn, L. *Vitamin E updated: new roles for the vitamin that preserves the health and integrity of body cells.* 26pp. 1983. New Canaan, Connecticut: Keats.

1618   Mervyn, L. *Vitamin E: the vitality vitamin.* 96pp. 1984. Wellingborough, Northamptonshire: Thorsons.
A comprehensive survey.

1619   Mervyn, L. *Vitamins A.D.K.* 96pp. 1984. Wellingborough, Northamptonshire: Thorsons.

1620   Mervyn, L. *The vitamins explained simply: all you need to know about vitamins, their sources and the effects they have on your health.* 128pp. 1984. Melbourne, Victoria: Science of Life Books.

1621   Mindell, Earl. *Pills and you.* 258pp. 1984. London: Arlington Books.
Looks at drugs and gives alternative natural remedies, vitamins, supplements and diets.

1622   Mindell, E. *Quick and easy guide to better health.* 118pp. 1982. New Canaan, Connecticut: Keats.
An instant reference to all important nutrients: vitamins, minerals and food supplements.

1623   Mindell, E. *The vitamin bible: how the right vitamins and minerals can revolutionize your life.* 213pp. 1983. London: Arlington Books.
One of the best all-round vitamin books.

1624   Mindell, E. *The vitamin bible for children.* 222pp. 1983. London: Arlington Books.
Informative and entertaining.

1625   Mindell, E. and William H. Lee. *The vitamin robbers: foods, drugs and pollutants that steal your nutrition.* 26pp. 1983. New Canaan, Connecticut: Keats.

1626 Mineral Laboratory Inc. (compilers). *A clinician's guide to toxic metals*. 23pp. 1979. Haywood, California: Mineral Laboratory.

1627 Mooney, Patrick. *The supernutrition handbook. A layman's guide to the new super health*. 142pp. 1981. San Francisco, California: By author. First published in 1978.

1628 Mount, J.L. *The food and health of Western man*. 270pp. 1979. Marlow, Buckinghamshire: Precision Press.

1629 National Advisory Committee on Nutrition Education. *A discussion paper on proposals for nutritional guidelines for health education in Britain*. 40pp. 1983. London: The Health Education Council.

1630 Newbold, H.L. *Meganutrients*. 360pp. 1975. New York: Peter H. Wyden.
Recommended.

1631 Newbold, H.L. *Vitamin C against cancer*. 363pp. 1979. New York: Stein and Day.
Reports on research findings.

1632 Norris, P.E. *About vitamins: nature's key to radiant health*. 64pp. 1982. Wellingborough, Northamptonshire: Thorsons.
A brief survey of the basic vitamins.

1633 Norris, P.E. *About wheat germ: nature's source of vital vitamins*. 63pp. 1980. Wellingborough, Northamptonshire: Thorsons.

1634 Nutrition Search Inc. (compilers). *Nutrition Almanac*. 279pp. 1979. New York: McGraw-Hill.

1635 Passwater, Richard A. *Cancer and its nutritional therapy*. 256pp. 1978. New Canaan, Connecticut: Keats.
A detailed discussion.

1636 Passwater, R.A. *Epa-marine lipids: in the battle against heart disease, an answer from the sea*. 26pp. 1982. New Canaan: Keats.

1637 Passwater, R.A. *Evening primrose oil: its amazing nutrients and the health benefits they can give you*. 30pp. 1981. New Canaan, Connecticut: Keats.

1638 Passwater, R.A. *G.T.F. chromium (glucose tolerance factor): its vitamin like properties could mean added protection against diabetes and heart disease.* 26pp. 1982. New Canaan, Connecticut: Keats.

1639   Passwater, R.A. *Selenium as food and medicine.* 240pp. 1980. New Canaan, Connecticut: Keats.

1640   Passwater, R.A. *Supernutrition.* 274pp. 1976. New York: Pocket Books.
    An excellent book.

1641   Passwater, R.A. *Supernutrition for healthy hearts.* 386pp. 1977. Wellingborough, Northamptonshire: Thorsons.

1642   Passwater, R.A. and Elmer M. Cranton. *Trace elements, hair analysis and nutrition.* 385pp. 1983. New Canaan, Connecticut: Keats.
    A major contribution to the field.

1643   Pauling, Linus C. *Vitamin C, the common cold and the flu.* 205pp. 1981. San Francisco, California: W.H. Freeman.
    An excellent, informative summary.

1644   Pauling, L.C. and Ewan Cameron. *Cancer and vitamin C: a discussion of the nature, causes, prevention and treatment of cancer with special references to the value of vitamin C.* 238pp. 1981. New York: Warner Books.
    Looks at orthodox treatment, its values and limitations as well as the use of vitamin C.

1645   Pfeiffer, Carl C. *Mental and elemental nutrients: a physician's guide to nutrition and health care.* 519pp. 1975. New Canaan, Connecticut: Keats.
    An in-depth discussion.

1646   Pfeiffer, C.C. *An updated fact book on zinc and other micronutrients.* 242pp. 1978. New Canaan, Connecticut: Keats.
    An informative guide.

1647   Pfeiffer, C.C. and Jane Banks. *Dr. Pfeiffer's total nutrition: eat well and stay well.* 161pp. 1982. London: Granada.
    A non-technical outline of Pfeiffer's orthomolecular approach.

1648   Philpott, William H. and Dwight K. Kalita. *Brain allergies: the psychonutrient connection.* 229pp. 1980. New Canaan, Connecticut: Keats.

1649 Philpott, W.H. and D.K. Kalita. *Victory over diabetes: a bio-ecologic triumph.* 294pp. 1983. New Canaan, Connecticut: Keats.
Looks at vitamins, minerals and diet.

1650 Plimmer, R.H.A. and Violet G. Plimmer. *Food, health and vitamins: being a new edition of food and health.* 120pp. 1929. London: Longmans, Greens and Co.

1651 Polunin, M. *Minerals: what they are and why we need them.* 96pp. 1982. Wellingborough, Northamptonshire: Thorsons.

1652 *Prevention* magazine (editors). *The complete book of vitamins.* 832pp. 1984. Emmaus, Pennsylvania: Rodale.

1653 *Prevention* magazine (editors). *Understanding vitamins and minerals.* 176pp. 1984. Emmaus, Pennsylvania: Rodale.
Describes how to make the best use of vitamins and minerals to keep healthy and fight disease.

1654 *Prevention* magazine (editors). *Vitamin A.* 130pp. 1972. Emmaus, Pennsylvania: Rodale.

1655 Randolph, Theron G. and Ralph W. Moss. *Allergies: your hidden enemy. How the new field of clinical ecology can unravel the environmental causes of mental and physical illness.* 70pp. 1983. Wellingborough, Northamptonshire: Thorsons.

1656 Randolph, T.G. and R.W. Moss. *An alternative approach to allergies.* 293pp. 1983. Wellingborough, Northamptonshire: Thorsons.
Recommended.

1657 Rippere, Vicky. *The allergy problem: why people suffer and what should be done.* 237pp. 1983. Wellingborough, Northamptonshire: Thorsons.
Looks at clinical ecology.

1658 Rippere, V. *Nutritional approaches to beahviour modification.* 55pp. 1983. New York: Academic Press.

1659 Rodale, J.I. and staff. *The complete book of minerals for health.* 813pp. n.d. Emmaus, Pennsylvania: Rodale.
A classic, but now out of date.

1660   Rodale, J.I. and staff (editors). *A complete guide to vitamins.* 319pp. 1968. Berkhamsted, Hertfordshire: Rodale.

1661   Rohé, Fred. *Metabolic ecology: a way to win the cancer war.* 237pp. 1982. Winfield, Kansas: Wedgestone Press.

1662   Rosenberg, Harold and A.N. Feldzamen. *The book of vitamin therapy: megavitamins for health.* 278pp. 1980. New York: G. Putman's Sons.
   Highly recommended.

1663   Ross, Harvey. *Fighting depression.* 221pp. 1975. New York: Larchmont Books.
   Megavitamins and special diets explained.

1664   Roth, June. *The food/depression connection: dietary control of allergy based mood swing.* 258pp. 1978. Chicago, Illinois: Contemporary Books.

1665   Royal College of Physicians. *Medical aspects of dietary fibre (a summary report of the Royal College of Physicians).* 175pp. 1981. London: Pitman Medical.

1666   Schroeder, Henry. *The poisons around us.* 144pp. 1978. New Canaan, Connecticut: Keats.
   Discusses metals and other elements as pollutants and as substances beneficial to life.

1667   Schroeder, H. *The trace elements of man.* 171pp. 1973. Old Greenwich, Connecticut: Devin-Adair.
   A serious book by a distinguished scientist.

1668   Science of Life Books (editors). *Heart ailments: their meaning, cause, and successful treatment.* 63pp. 1980. Melbourne, Victoria: Science of Life Books.
   Explains the vitamin E therapy.

1669   Science Publishing House (editors). *Vitamin B_{15} (pangamic acid): properties, functions and use.* 205pp. 1965. Los Angeles, California: Cancer Book House.
   A translation of various studies carried out in the USSR.

1670   Scott, Cyril. *Crude black molasses: nature's wonder food.* 48pp. 1978. Wellingborough, Northamptonshire: Thorsons.
   Describes this source of important nutrients.

1671 Shears, C. Curtis. *Orthomolecular nutrition: the science of self-healing*. 95pp. 1980. Gloucester: The Nutritional Science Research Institute.

1672 Sherman, Henry C. *The science of nutrition*. 253pp. 1944. Oxford University Press. London: Humphrey Milford.

1673 Shroeder, H.A. *The trace elements and man*. 786pp. 1972. San Francisco, California: W.H. Freeman.

1674 Shute, Evan V. *Common questions on vitamin E and their answers*. 100pp. 1979. New Canaan, Connecticut: Keats.

1675 Shute, E.V. *The heart and vitamin E*. 148pp. 1977. New Canaan, Connecticut: Keats.

1676 Shute, Wilfred E. *Complete updated vitamin E book*. 255pp. 1978. New Canaan, Connecticut: Keats.

1677 Shute, W.V. *Health preserver: defining the versatility of vitamin E*. 167pp. 1977. Emmaus, Pennsylvania: Rodale.

1678 Shute, W.V. *Your child and vitamin E*. 153pp. 1979. New Canaan, Connecticut: Keats.

1679 Shute, W.V. with Harold J. Taub. *Vitamin E for ailing and healthy hearts*. 208pp. 1971. London: W.A. Allen.

1680 Simons, Paul. *Lecithin: the cholesterol controller*. 96pp. 1983. Wellingborough, Northamptonshire: Thorsons.

1681 Stone, Irwin. *The healing factor: vitamin C against disease*. 258pp. 1979. New York: Grosset and Dunlap.
A definitive book on vitamin C.

1682 Sullivan, George. *Additives in your food*. 128pp. 1976. New York: Simon and Schuster.
A dictionary of the most common additives. Simple to read.

1683 Timms, Moira and Zachariah Zar. *Natural sources: vitamin B_{17}/laetrile*. 149pp. 1978. Millbrae, California: Celestial Arts.
A useful and practical guide to vitamin B_{17}, its natural sources and role in cancer prevention. For the layman.

1684   Truss, C. Orian. *The missing diagnosis*. 165pp. 1982. Birmingham, Alabama: C. Orian Truss.
Clinical papers on human illness caused by *Candida albicans*.

1685   Wade, Carlson. *Carlson Wade's lecithin book: what you need to know*. 112pp. 1980. New Canaan, Connecticut: Keats.

1686   Wade, C. *Carlson Wade's vitamins, minerals and other supplements*. 148pp. 1983. New Canaan, Connecticut: Keats.

1687   Wade, C. *Magic minerals*. 229pp. 1972. New York: Arco.
A review.

1688   Wade, C. *The miracle of organic vitamins for better health*. 255pp. 1979. West Nyack, New York: Parker Publishing Company.

1689   Wade, C. *The rejuvenation vitamin (vitamin E)*. 188pp. 1970. London: Tandem Books.

1690   Wade, C. *Vitamins and other food supplements and your health*. 119pp. 1974. New Canaan, Connecticut: Keats.
A useful, brief guide.

1691   Watson, George. *Nutrition and your mind*. 204pp. 1980. New York: Bantam Books.
A popular book.

1692   Wentzler, Rich. *The vitamin book*. 257pp. 1978. New York: St. Martin's Press.
A comprehensive and readable analysis.

1693   Williams, Roger J. *Nutrition against disease*. 370pp. 1981. New York: Bantam Books.
Recommended.

1694   Williams, R.J. *A physician's handbook of nutritional science*. 127pp. 1977. Elmsford, New York: Pergamon Press.
Reviews the orthomolecular field.

1695   Williams, R.J. and Dwight K. Kalita. *Physician's handbook on orthomolecular medicine*. 207pp. 1979. New Canaan, Connecticut: Keats.
A definitive collection of articles and papers on orthomolecular medicine.

1696   Wright, Jonathan V. *Dr. Wright's book of nutritional therapy: real-life lessons in medicine without drugs.* 529pp. 1979. Emmaus, Pennsylvania: Rodale.
Vitamin and mineral therapy.

1697   Wright, J.V. *Dr. Wright's guide to healing with nutrition.* 624pp. 1984. Emmaus, Pennsylvania: Rodale.
Healing body and mind without drugs or survery using vitamins and minerals.

Osteopathy

1698   Arbuckle, Beryl E. *The selected writings of Beryl E. Arbuckle.* 264pp. n.d. Newark, Ohio: American Academy of Osteopathy.
  Looks at cranial osteopathy.

1699   Ashmore, Edythe F. *Osteopathic mechanics: a textbook.* 237pp. 1981. London: Tamor Pierston Publishers.

1700   Barber, Elmer D. *Osteopathy complete.* 572pp. 1906. Kansas City, Missouri: Franklin Hudson. First published in 1898.

1701   Barker, Herbert. *Leaves from my life.* 319pp. 1927. London: Hutchinson.
  Letters and papers relating to attitudes of orthodoxy and political problems relating to Barker's practising with an osteopath.

1702   Bennett, George Matthews. *Art of the bone-setter: a testimony and a vindication.* 144pp. 1981. London: Tamor Pierston. First published in 1884.

1703   Bigsby, Myron H. *Osteopathic diagnosis and technique with chapters on osteopathic landmarks.* 262pp. 1907. Vineland, New Jersey: Commercial Printing House.

1704   Blum, S. *Paediatric symptomology and differential diagnosis.* 500pp. 1938. Name of publisher not given.
  Excellent sections on osteopathy.

1705   Booth, E.R. *History of osteopathy and 20th century medical practice.* 835pp. 1924. Cincinnati, Ohio: By author.
  Perhaps the most comprehensive history of osteopathy.

1706   British School of Osteopathy, The. *The British School of Osteopathy Diamond Jubilee Year Book*. 74pp. 1977. London: The British School of Osteopathy.

1707   Brookes, Denis. *Lectures on cranial osteopathy: a manual for practitioners and students*. 144pp. 1981. Wellingborough, Northamptonshire: Thorsons.
   A guide to the principles, practice and benefits of cranial bone manipulation.

1708   Burns, L. *Studies in the osteopathic sciences*. Volume 1: *Basic principles*. Volume 2: *The nerve centers*. Volume 3: *The physiology of consciousness*. Volume 4: *The blood*. All over 300 pages long. 1911. Cincinnati, Ohio: Monfort.
   Of historical interest. Volume 3 is still of use today.

1709   Burton, A.K. *A work study of the Osteopathic Association of Great Britain: the characteristics of patients*. 1977. London: The Osteopathic Association of Great Britain.

1710   Burton, J. Guymer (compiler). *Osteopathy explained: what is osteopathy, what does it do?* 36pp. 1974. Privately published by author.

1711   Campbell, Giraud. *A doctor's proven new home cure for arthritis*. 224pp. 1972. Englewood Cliffs, New Jersey: Prentice-Hall.
   Written by an osteopath who combines manipulation and pure foods in his treatment for arthritis.

1712   Canning, James. *Osteopathy: a basic science*. 20pp. 1956. Printed for the British School of Osteopathy.

1713   Castlio, Yale (editor). *Collected papers of Dr. George J. Canley*. 432pp. 1935. Kansas City, Missouri: The Kansas City College of Osteopathy and Surgery.

1714   Castilio, Y. *Principles of osteopathy*. 311pp. n.d. Kansas City, Missouri: The Kansas City College of Osteopathy and Surgery.
   Was a useful book when it was written (in the 1940s).

1715   Cayce, J. Gail. *Osteopathy*. 64pp. 1973. Virginia Beach, Virginia: ARE Press.
   A comparison of various parallel concepts expressed by A.T. Still and Edgar Cayce.

1716   Chaitow, Leon. *Osteopathy: a complete health care system: an explanation of the concept of osteopathy and the potentials of osteopathic treatment.* 112pp. 1983. Wellingborough, Northamptonshire: Thorsons.

1717   Chaitow, L. *Osteopathy: head-to-toe health through manipulation.* 92pp. 1979. Wellingborough, Northamptonshire: Thorsons.
Explains the origins of osteopathy and its development as well as reviewing the latest trends in osteopathic research and training.

1718   Chesterton, Mrs Cecil. *This thy body: an experience in osteopathy.* 160pp. n.d. London: Stanley Paul.
Written at the time of the 1935 Lords Select Committee on Osteopathy, this book looks at the history of osteopathy and puts the case for it.

1719   Christensen, K.D. *Extremity adjusting.* 34pp. 1978. Portland, Oregon: Copy Break Printing.

1720   Clark, Marion Edward. *Applied anatomy: designed for the use of osteopathic students and practitioners as an aid in the anatomical explanation of disease from an osteopathic viewpoint.* 687pp. 1906. Kirksville, Missouri: The Journal Printing Co.

1721   Clark, M.E. *Diseases of women: a manual of gynecology designed for the use of osteopathic students and practitioners.* 1901. 378pp. Kirksville, Missouri: Democrat Print.
Excellent.

1722   Committee of Inquiry into Chiropractic, Osteopathy, Homoeopathy and Naturopathy. *Report of the Committee of Inquiry into Chiropractic, Osteopathy, Homoeopathy and Naturopathy.* 925pp. 1977. Canberra, Australia: Australian Government Publishing Service.
Looks at alternative health care in Australia.

1723   Conti, Gustave V. *Structural analysis: osteopathic manipulative management of spine and extremities.* 154pp. 1975. Privately published by author.
This is a good example of recent U.S. osteopathic teaching specifically relating to the manipulative aspect of American osteopathy.

1724   Curry, Etna K. and Byron H. Comstock. *Osteopathy in abstract.* 167pp. 1926. Name of publisher not given.
A useful reference book for the practitioner and student.

1725   Cyriax, James. *Osteopathy and manipulation*. 92pp. 1949. London: Crosby Lockwood and Son.
   Argues against osteopathy.

1726   Darlison, J.J. *The new art of healing: osteopathy. Some popular questions answered*. 46pp. n.d. Privately published by author.
   For the general reader of the 1930s.

1727   Davis, A.P. *Osteopathy illustrated: a drugless system of healing*. 851pp. 1899. Cincinnati, Ohio: Fred L. Rowe.

1728   Deason, J. *Diseases of the head and neck*. 243pp. 1921. Kirksville, Missouri: The Journal Printing Co.
   Presents the osteopathic concept as applied to the treatment of the head and neck. For the practitioner and student.

1729   Deason, J. *On the osteopathic treatment of diseases of the ear, nose and throat*. 128pp. 1915. Bulletin Number 3. Chicago, Illinois: The A.T. Still Research Institute.

1730   Deason, J. *Physiology: general and osteopathic: a reference and text book for practitioners and students*. 586pp. 1913. Kirksville, Missouri: The Journal Printing Co.

1731   Deason, J. *Research in osteopathy*. 223pp. 1916. Bulletin Number 2. Chicago, Illinois: The A.T. Still Research Institute.

1732   Devon, David. *Hands for healing*. 159pp. 1966. London: Corgi.
   A book for the general reader.

1733   Dove, Colin I. *A history of the Osteopathic Association of Great Britain*. 16pp. n.d. London: Osteopathic Association of Great Britain. (Reprinted from the *British Osteopathic Journal*, vol. 3, no. 3, 1967).

1734   Downing, Carter Harrison. *Osteopathic principles in diseases*. 623pp. 1935. San Francisco: Ricardo J. Orozco.
   Recommended.

1735   Downing, C.H. *Principles and practice of osteopathy*. 402pp. 1981. London: Tamor Pierston.
   Originally published in 1923.

1736   Downing, C.H. *Simplified spinal technique*. 50pp. n.d. Boston, Massachusetts: Massachusetts College of Osteopathy. Reprinted for the use of students in the Department of Osteopathic Technique, Massachusetts College of Osteopathy.

1737   Drew, Ira W. (editor). *The osteopathic treatment of children's diseases*. 823pp. 1923. Los Angeles, California: The A.T. Still Research Institute. Produced by the education department.

1738   Dummer, Thomas G. *Osteopathic technique*. 5pp. 1981. Maidstone, Kent: The European School of Osteopathy.

1739   Dummer, T.G. *The 'unregistered' practitioner and the law*. 40pp. n.d. Maidstone, Kent: The European School of Osteopathy.

1740   Dunning, Muriel Higham. *Osteopathy and the development of the vertebral column*. 32pp. 1959. London: The Osteopathic Publishing Co.
   Lecture given as 'the John Martin Littlejohn Memorial Lecture' in 1959.

1741   Ellis, A.W. *First steps in osteopathy*. 32pp. n.d. London: The Osteopathic Publishing Co.

1742   European College of Osteopathy. *The mechanics of the spine and pelvis*. 17pp. 1983. Maidstone, Kent: European College of Osteopathy.
   Articles derived from the 1956 *Maidstone Institute of Applied Technique Year Book*.

1743   Feyette, Harrison H. *Principles of osteopathic technic*. 246pp. 1980. Colorado Springs, Colorado: The American Academy of Osteopathy.
   A classic work of the early 1950s. When it was first published in 1954 Feyette gave a copy of his book to each registered osteopath.

1744   Foote, Harvey. *The science of osteopathy*. 15pp. 1927. Privately published by author.

1745   Fowler, L.N. and Co. (compiled for). *A home study course in osteopathy, massage and manual therapeutics*. 130pp. 1914. London: L.N. Fowler.
   A curiosity. Parts of this book are copied wholesale from *Osteopathy complete* by Elmer D. Barber (1898).

1746   General Council and Register of Osteopaths, The. *Code of ethics*.

159

22pp. n.d. London: The General Council and Register of Osteopaths. Compiled in the 1980s.

1747 General Council and Register of Osteopaths, The. *The osteopathic blue book: the origins and development of osteopathy in Great Britain.* 78pp. n.d. London: General Council and Register of Osteopaths.
A nice book but out of date.

1748 Gillett, Clyde F. *The Gillett course in eye, ear, nose and throat.* Pages unnumbered. 1931. Los Angeles, California: By author.

1749 Goetz, Edward W. *A manual of osteopathy with the application of physical cultures, baths and diet.* 177pp. 1905. Cincinnati, Ohio: By author.

1750 Goldthwaite, Joel E., Lloyd T. Brown, Loring T. Swaim, John G. Kuhns. *Essentials of body mechanics in health and disease.* 356pp. 1945. Philadelphia, Pennsylvania: J.B. Lippincott Co.

1751 Gour, Andrew A. *Therapeutics of activity.* 478pp. 1923. Chicago, Illinois: Covici-McGee.
A classic, originally published in 1916.

1752 Grasset, Hector (translated by Jocelyn C. Proby). *Bechamp: An appreciation (L'Oeuvre de Bechamp).* 119pp. n.d. Maidstone, Kent: Osteopathic Institute of Applied Technique. First French edition was published in 1913.

1753 Gregory, Alva. *Spinal adjustment technique.* 565pp. n.d. O'Fallon, Missouri: W.G. Bazan.

1754 Grow, O.P. *Osteopathic obstetrics.* 94pp. 1933. Queen City, Missouri: The Journal Printing Co.

1755 Hall, T. Edward and John Wernham. *The contribution of John Martin Littlejohn to osteopathy.* 81pp. 1978. Maidstone, Kent: Maidstone Osteopathic Clinic.
Inaugural address to 'the John Martin Littlejohn Memorial lecture' in 1952.

1756 Halladay, H.V. (edited by A.C. Walmsley). *Applied anatomy of the spine.* 205pp. 1920. Kirksville, Missouri: J.F. Janisch.
Anatomy for osteopaths.

1757   Hartman, Laurie S. *Handbook of osteopathic technique*. 204pp. 1983. Hertfordshire: N.M.K.
One of the best books on osteopathic technique.!?!

1758   Haycock, Willis. *The expanding concept of osteopathy*. 35pp. 1955. London: The Osteopathic Publishing Co.
Given as 'the John Martin Littlejohn Memorial Lecture' in 1955.

1759   Hazzard, Charles. *Practice and applied therapeutics of osteopathy*. 442pp. 1905. Kirksville, Missouri: The Journal Printing Co.
Was the standard textbook of the day and is still of use today.

1760   Hazzard, Charles. *Principles of osteopathy*. 319pp. 1899. Kirksville, Missouri: Name of publisher not given. The 1891 edition was in two volumes and included five chapters not found in this edition.

1761   Henderson, John J. *Spinal adjustment and mechanical treatment*. 149pp. 1922. Charles Town, West Virginia: Name of publisher not given.
A simply written text.

1762   Henry, Eugene Howe. *Sexual hygiene (from an osteopathic viewpoint): a scientific discussion of physiological and pathological sexual relations*. 141pp. n.d. Kirksville, Missouri: Printed for private distribution.
A series of twelve lectures personally revised from stenographic reports. A curiosity.

1763   Hildreth, Arthur Grant. *The lengthening shadow of Dr. Andrew Taylor Still*. 457pp. 1942. Macon, Missouri: Mrs. A.G. Hildreth, and Paw Paw, Michigan: Mrs. A.E. Van Vleck.
Recommended.

1764   Hilton, John. *Rest and pain: a course of lectures on the influence of mechanical and physiological rest in the treatment of accidents and surgical diseases and the diagnostic value of pain*. 511pp. 1880. London: George Bell and Sons.
A classic Victorian text, not osteopathic, but one that influenced osteopathic thinking and treatment.

1765   Hoag, J. Marshall, Wilbur V. Cole and Spencer G. Bradford (editors). *Osteopathic medicine*. 786pp. 1969. New York: McGraw-Hill.
Provides an integrated view of present rationale and practice in the field of osteopathy.

1766   Hollis, A.S. *The principles of osteopathic technique*. 112pp. 1914. Kirksville, Missouri: AMS.

1767   Hood, Wharton P. *A` treatise on bone-setting*. 156pp. 1871. London: Macmillan.

1768   Horler, Sydney. *I accuse the doctors: being a candid commentary on the hostility shown by the leaders of the medical profession towards the healing art of osteopathy, and how the public suffer in consequence*. 147pp. 1949. London: Alvin Redman.

1769   Hulett, G.D. *A textbook of the principles of osteopathy*. 179pp. 1922. Kirksville, Missouri: The A.T. Still Research Institute.
An excellent reference book. This edition, known as 'Hulett's Principles', has been extensively revised by various committees and is much slimmer than the first edition (1903: 366pp).

1770   Incorporated Association of Osteopathy, The. *Osteopathy: what it is*. 15pp. n.d. Issued by the authority of the Incorporated Association of Osteopathy Ltd.

1771   Jarnette, Bertrand De. *Cranial technique*. 240pp. 1979. Nebraska City, Nebraska: By author.
A textbook.

1772   Jones, Lawrence H. *Strain and counterstrain*. 111pp. 1981. Colorado Springs, Colorado: The American Academy of Osteopathy.
Recommended.

1773   Journal of the Society of Osteopaths. *Osteopathy and health care*. 28pp. n.d. London: Journal of the Society of Osteopaths.

1774   Keesecker, Raymond P. *The osteopathic movement in medicine: a source document*. 1957. Chicago, Illinois: The American Osteopathic Association.

1775   Kent Rush, Anne. *The basic back book*. 254pp. 1980. London: Wildwood House.

1776   Korr, Irvin M. *The physiological basis of osteopathic medicine*. 116pp. 1975. New York: The Postgraduate Institute of Osteopathic Medicine and Surgery.
Written by a physiologist.

1777   Kugelmass, I. Newton (editor). *The physiologic basis of osteopathic medicine.* 116pp. 1970. New York: The Postgraduate Institute of Osteopathic Medicine and Surgery.
Adapted from a symposium presented on 7 October 1967.

1778   Lane, M.A. *Dr. A.T. Still: founder of osteopathy.* 218pp. 1925. Waukegan, Illinois: The Bunting Publications.
An appreciation of Still's work and contribution to osteopathy.

1779   Laughlin, Earl Herbert. *Quiz on the practice of osteopathy: compendium of ready reference for the busy practitioner and advanced student.* 137pp. 1903. Kirksville, Missouri: By author.

1780   Laughlin, Geo. M. *et al. Case reports from Kirksville Osteopathic Hospitals.* 219pp. n.d. Kirksville, Missouri: Kirksville Osteopathic Hospitals.

1781   Laughlin, William Ross. *Anatomy in a nutshell: a treatise on human anatomy in its relation to osteopathy.* 616pp. n.d. Kirksville, Missouri: By author.
Excellent.

1782   Laycock, Byron E. *Manual of joint manipulation.* 431pp. 1953. Des Moines, Iowa: Still College of Osteopathy.
One of the first textbooks to make extensive use of photographic material to demonstrate osteopathic technique.

1783   Lindlahr, Henry. *Natural therapeutics: philosophy of natural therapeutics.* Volume 1. 327pp. 1975. Maidstone, Kent: The Maidstone Osteopathic Clinic. First published in 1926.

1784   Lindlahr, H. *Natural therapeutics: practice of natural therapeutics.* Volume 2. 312pp. 1981. Saffron Walden, Essex: C.W. Daniel. First published in 1919.

1785   Lippincott, Rebecca C. and Howard A. Lippincott. *A manual of cranial technique.* 101pp. n.d. Privately published by authors.

1786   Littlejohn, James B. *Notes on histology.* 70pp. 1899. St. Louis, Missouri: Becktold Printing and Publishing Co.

1787   Littlejohn, J.B. *The outlines of pathology.* 124pp. Kirksville, Missouri: Weekly Advocate Print.

1788   Littlejohn, John Martin. *The fundamentals of osteopathic technique.* 291pp. n.d. Maidstone, Kent: The Maidstone Osteopathic Clinic.

1789   Littlejohn, J.M. *Lecture notes on physiology: delivered before the January and April classes of the American School of Osteopathy.* 277pp. 1898. Kirksville, Missouri: Advocate Book and Job Print.

1790   Littlejohn, J.M. *Lectures on psycho-physiology.* 163pp. 1899. Kirksville, Missouri: The American School of Osteopathy.

1791   Littlejohn, J.M. *Notes on the principle of osteopathy.* 34pp. n.d. Maidstone, Kent: The Maidstone Osteopathic Clinic.

1792   Littlejohn, J.M. *Osteopathy: lectures on pathology.* 112pp. n.d. Maidstone, Kent: The Maidstone Osteopathic Clinic.

1793   Littlejohn, J.M. *Physiology: exhaustive and practical.* Part II. 832pp. n.d. Name of publisher not given.

1794   Littlejohn, J.M. and Lawrence S. Meyran. *Practice of osteopathy.* Volume 1. 433pp. n.d. Name of publisher not given.

1795   Littlejohn, J.M. and L.S. Meyran. *Principles of osteopathy.* 432pp. n.d. Chicago, Illinois: Name of publisher not given.

1796   Litton, Harold E. and the staff of the Department of Osteopathic Technique of the College of Osteopathic Physicians and Surgeons in Los Angeles. *Handbook of osteopathic technique.* 153pp. 1944. Los Angeles, California: The College of Osteopathic Physicians and Surgeons.
    Still a useful technique book.

1797   Lowenkopf, Anne N. *Osteopuncture: relief from strong and chronic pain.* 196pp. 1976. Santa Barbara, California: Medical Arts.
    Describes what osteopuncture is, and what it can do.

1798   Lowry, Gerald. *A place among men.* 73pp. 1928. London: Mondiale.
    Written by a blind osteopath.

1799   Lowry, G. *From Mons to 1933.* 133pp. 1934. London: Simpkin Marshall, Hamilton, Kent and Co. Ltd.
    Describes how the author trained to be an osteopath despite being blind.

1800   Lowry, G. *Helping hands.* 128pp. 1935. London: John Lane The Bodley Head.
Sets out to show how osteopathy can help in many different cases of ill health.

1801   McCole, George Malcolm. *An analysis of the osteopathic lesion: A study in pathology, physiology and anatomy.* 344pp. 1935. Great Falls, Montana: Geo. M. McCole, D.O., Publisher.
A great milestone in the development of osteopathic thinking.

1802   McConnell, Carl Philip (editor). *Clinical osteopathy.* 643pp. 1917. Chicago, Illinois: The A.T. Still Research Institute.
Many interesting treatments for various conditions, comprehensively listed.

1803   McConnell, C.P. *Notes on osteopathic therapeutics.* 237pp. 1898. Kirksville, Missouri: The Journal Printing Co.

1804   McConnell, C.P. and Charles Clayton Teall. *The practice of osteopathy.* 807pp. 1920. Kirksville, Missouri: The Journal Printing Co. Originally written by McConnell in 1899. First edition by McConnell and Teall was in 1906.
For the practitioner and student.

1805   MacDonald, George and W. Hargrave-Wilson. *The osteopathic lesion.* 141pp. 1935. London: William Heinemann.
An important book in the history of the principles of osteopathy, and still of use today.

1806   Macdonald, W. Kelman *et al. Report on the scientific basis of osteopathy.* 367pp. 1935. Name of publisher not given.
A report based on the seven bulletins of the A.T. Still Research Institute and on other selected contributions to the *Journal of the American Osteopathic Association* by various osteopathic research workers. It was presented to the Select Committee of the House of Lords on Registration and Regulation of the Osteopaths Bill.

1807   Magoun, Harold I. *Osteopathy in the cranial field: the application to the cranium of the principles of osteopathy, based on the arduous study and keen clinical observation of William Garner Sutherland.* 367pp. 1976. Meridian, Idaho: The Cranial Academy. First published in 1966.

1808   Maidstone Osteopathic Clinic, The. *Mechanics of the spine and pelvis.* Maidstone, Kent: The Maidstone Osteopathic Clinic.

1809   Matthay, Ferdinand L. *The cure of disease by osteopathy, hydropathy and hygiene: A book for the people giving directions for the treatment and cure of diseases without the use of drug medicine.* 96pp. 1900. Privately published by author.
   Of historical interest.

1810   McKeon, L.C. Floyd. *A healing crisis.* 175pp. 1933. Weston-super-Mare, Avon: Michell Health Products.
   Looks at osteopathy, chiropractic and naturopathy.

1811   McKeon, L.C.F. *Osteopathy and Chiropractic explained.* 108pp. 1927. London: Lutterworth Press.

1812   McKeon, L.C.F. *Osteopathic polemics.* 158pp. 1938. London: C.W. Daniel.

1813   McManis, J.V. *Unitary technic: The technic of integration, correlation and reciprocal action.* Pages not numbered. 1938. Kirksville, Missouri: Morrow-McManis.

1814   Mellor, Ethel. *Manipulation as a curative factor: osteopathy and medicine, with an appendix on hay fever.* 255pp. 1931. London: Methuen.

1815   Mennell, James. *Backache.* 227pp. 1935. Philadelphia, Pennsylvania: P. Blakiston's Sons.

1816   Mennell, J. *The science and art of joint manipulation.* Volume I: *The extremities.* 215pp. 1949. Volume II: *The spinal column.* 264pp. 1952. Philadelphia, Pennsylvania: The Blakiston Company.

1817   Middleton, H.C. *Osteopathy and visceral disease.* 14pp. 1957. London: The British School of Osteopathy.
   Given as 'the John Martin Littlejohn Memorial Lecture' in 1957.

1818   Millard, E.P. (edited by A.G. Walmsley). *Applied anatomy of the lymphatics.* 276pp. 1922. Kirksville, Missouri: The Journal Printing Co.

1819   Millard, F.P. *Practical visions: a book of inspiration.* 270pp. 1922. Kirksville, Missouri: The Journal Printing Co.

1820   Mitchell, Fred L., Peter S. Morn and Neil A. Pruzzo. *An evaluation and treatment manual of osteopathic muscle energy procedures.* 565pp. 1980. Manchester, Missouri: By authors.
   Recommended.

1821   Moulton, Friar. *The complete bone-setter.* Pages not numbered. 1981. Isleworth, Middlesex: Tamor Pierston. Originally published in 1656.

1822   Murray, Chas. H. *Practice of osteopathy: its practical application to the various diseases of the human body.* 412pp. 1918. Elgin, Illinois: Name of publisher not given.
   A classic.

1823   Murray, C.H. and M.S. Murray. *A drugless treatment for partial deafness and deafness: osteopathic, somapathic, naturopathic, chiropractic, mechanotherapic.* 40pp. 1915. Elgin, Illinois: The Murray Publishers.

1824   Murray, C.H. and M.S. Murray. *Osteopathic gynecology: a textbook on the diseases of women with the appropriate treatment from the drugless standpoint.* 196pp. 1915. Elgin, Illinois: The Murray Publishers.

1825   Nicholas, N.S. *Atlas of osteopathic techniques.* 71pp. 1980. Philadelphia, Pennsylvania: By author and The Philadelphia College of Osteopathic Medicine.
   An excellent textbook on technique.

1826   Northrup, George W. *Osteopathic medicine: an American reformation.* 87pp. 1979. Chicago, Illinois: The American Osteopathic Association.
   An overview.

1827   Osteopaths Bill, The. *A report of the proceedings before a select committee of the House of Lords.* 1935.

1828   Page, Leon E. *The old doctor.* 45pp. 1932. Kirksville, Missouri: The Journal of Osteopathy.

1829   Page, L.E. *Osteopathic fundamentals.* 182pp. 1981. London: Tamor Pierston.

1830   Page, L.E. *The principles of osteopathy.* 292pp. 1952. Kansas City, Missouri: The Academy of Applied Osteopathy.
   Recommended.

1831   Peterson, Barbara (editor). *The collected papers of Irvin M. Korr.*

256pp. 1979. Colorado Springs, Colorado: The American Academy of Osteopathy.
Recommended.

1832   Peterson, B. (editor). *Postural balance and imbalance.* 159pp. 1983. Newark, Ohio: The American Academy of Osteopathy.
A selection of papers from the yearbooks on these subjects.

1833   Postgraduate Institute of Osteopathic Medicine and Surgery (edited by). *The physiological basis of osteopathic medicine.* 116pp. 1975. New York: Insight Publications.
Includes papers by five contributors.

1834   Proby, Jocelyn C. *Essays on osteopathy: its principles, application and scope.* 44pp. 1955. Maidstone, Kent: The Osteopathic Institute of Applied Technique. Originally printed in 1937 for private circulation.

1835   Proby, J.C. *The place of osteopathy in therapeutics.* 34pp. 1953. London: The Osteopathic Publishing Co.
Given as 'the John Martin Littlejohn Memorial Lecture' in 1953.

1836   Riggs, Wilfred. *A manual of osteopathic manipulation and treatment.* 157pp. 1901. Elkhart, Indiana: New Science Publishing Co.

1837   Riggs, W. *Theory of osteopathy.* 218pp. 1900. Des Moines, Iowa: New Science Publishing Co.

1838   Romer, Frank. *Modern bone-setting for the medical profession.* 77pp. 1915. London: William Heinemann.

1839   Rubinstein, Samuel H. (editor). *Osteopathic techniques.* 72pp. 1949. Philadelphia, Pennsylvania: Louis J. Marks.
A book for the general reader.

1840   Smith, Audrey E. *Osteopathic diagnosis.* 51pp. 1984. London: The British School of Osteopathy.
For students of the School.

1841   Smith, Oakley. *Connective tissue cause of disease: naprapathic connectivology.* 40pp. 1919. Chicago: Chicago College of Naprapathy.

1842   Still, Andrew Taylor. *Autobiography of A.T. Still.* 460pp. 1897. Kirksville, Missouri: By author.
Very interesting reading.

1843   Still, A.T. *Osteopathy, research and practice.* 53pp. 1910. Kirksville, Missouri: By author.
Probably Still's most useful work.

1844   Still, A.T. *The philosophy of osteopathy.* 268pp. 1977. Colorado Springs, Colorado: The American Academy of Osteopathy. First published in 1899.

1845   Still, A.T. *Philosophy and mechanical principles of osteopathy.* 319pp. 1902. Kansas City, Missouri: Hudson-Kimberley. First published 1892.

1846   A.T. Still Research Institute, The (editors). *Changes in the body fluids due to vertebral lesions.* 199pp. 1931. Bulletin Number 7. Chicago, Illinois: The A.T. Still Research Institute.

1847   A.T. Still Research Institute, The (editors). *A contribution to the study of the pathology of the vertebral lesion.* 185pp. 1917. Bulletin Number 4. Chicago, Illinois: The A.T. Still Research Institute.

1848   A.T. Still Research Institute, The (editors). *Further contributions to the study of the effects of lumbar lesions.* 185pp. 1917. Bulletin Number 5. Chicago, Illinois: The A.T. Still Research Institute.

1849   A.T. Still Research Institute, The (editors). *The A.T. Still Research Institute.* 63pp. 1910. Bulletin Number 1. Chicago, Illinois: The A.T. Still Research Institute.

1850   A.T. Still Research Institute, The (editors). *A study of certain growth changes due to vertebral lesions in rabbits and other mammals: miscellaneous papers.* 123pp. 1926. Bulletin Number 6. Chicago, Illinois: The A.T. Still Research Institute.

1851   Stoddard, Alan. *The back: relief from pain. Patterns of back pain, how to deal with and avoid them.* 125pp. 1980. London: Martin Dunitz.
Contains practical hints and simple exercises.

1852   Stoddard, A. *Manual of osteopathic practice.* 350pp. 1983. London: Hutchinson.
A companion to the author's *Manual of osteopathic technique.*

1853   Stoddard, A. *Manual of osteopathic technique.* 275pp. 1980. London: Hutchinson.
Of great value to professionals in the field.

1854 Straten, L. van. *About your low back.* 8pp. n.d. London: The Osteopathic Association of Great Britain.

1855 Streeter, Wilfred A. *The new healing.* 257pp. 1932. London: Methuen.
Streeter was in favour of a select committee on osteopathy and this book was a political statement.

1856 Sutherland, Adah S. *With thinking fingers: the story of William Garner Sutherland.* 98pp. 1962. Kansas City, Missouri: The Cranial Academy.

1857 Sutherland, A. Strand and Anne L. Wales (assembled and edited by). *Collected writings of William Garner Sutherland, D.O., D.Sc. (Hons): pertaining to the art and science of osteopathy including the cranial concept on osteopathy.* 254pp. 1967. Produced under the auspices of the Sutherland Cranial Teaching Foundation.

1858 Sutherland, William Garner (edited and assembled by Adah Strand Sutherland). *Contributions of thought.* 54pp. 1967. Produced under the auspices of the Sutherland Cranial Teaching Foundation. No address given.

1859 Sutherland, W.G. *The cranial bowl: A treatise relating to cranial articular mobility, cranial articular lesions and cranial technic.* 140pp. 1948. Mankato, Minnesota: By author.

1860 Swart, Joseph. *Osteopathic strap technic.* 179pp. 1923. Kansas City, Missouri: Joseph Swart.
A useful and interesting book first published in 1919.

1861 Tasker, Dain L. *Principles of osteopathy.* 589pp. 1925. Los Angeles: Bireley and Elson Printing Co.
An excellent osteopathic text comprehensively covering all aspects of the subject.

1862 Truhlar, Robert E. *Doctor A.T. Still in the living.* 154pp. 1950. Chagrin Falls, Ohio: By author.
Recommended.

1863 Tucker, Ernest Eckford. *Osteopathic technic.* 174pp. 1917. New York: Clinton Press.
A clear, succinct account.

1864 Tucker, E.E. and Perrin T. Wilson. *The theory of osteopathy.* 96pp. 1936. Privately published by authors.
A stimulating dissertation on the philosophy of osteopathy.

1865 Upledger, John E. and Jon D. Vredevoogd. *Craniosacral therapy.* 367pp. 1983. Chicago, Illinois: Eastland Press.
Defines the physiology and anatomy of the craniosacral system, its function in health and its relationship to disease processes. The best textbook on the subject.

1866 Walton, William J. *Textbook of osteopathic diagnosis and technique procedures.* 547pp. 1970. Colorado Springs, Colorado: The American Academy of Osteopathy. Originally published as *A manual of osteopathic technic* in 1945.
An account of osteopathy in the United States.

1867 Webster, George V. *Concerning osteopathy: a compilation of selections from articles published in the professional and lay press with original chapters.* 242pp. 1919. Norward, Massachusetts: The Plimpton Press.

1868 Webster, G.V. *Sage sayings of Still.* 1935. Los Angeles, California: Wetzel.

1869 Webster, G.V. *Something wrong.* 88pp. 1918. Norward, Massachusetts: The Plimpton Press.

1870 Webster-Jones, S. *Osteopathy as revealed in writings of Andrew Taylor Still.* 33pp. 1954. London: The British School of Osteopathy.

1871 Wernham, John (editor). *The fundamentals of osteopathic technique. Edited writings of J.M. Littlejohn.* 293pp. 1983. Maidstone, Kent: Maidstone Osteopathic Clinic.

1872 Wernham, J. (edited and revised by). *Osteopathy: notes on the technique and practice.* 116pp. 1975. Maidstone, Kent: The Maidstone Osteopathic Clinic.
Recommended.

1873 Wernham, J. *The philosophy and mechanics of osteopathy.* 23pp. n.d. Maidstone, Kent: The Maidstone Osteopathic Clinic.
The content comes from an address given before the members of the Association Française des Ostéopathes at the first European Congress held in Paris on 18 November 1978.

1874   Wernham, J. and Mervyn Waldman. *An illustrated manual of osteopathic technique*. Volume 1: 304pp. 1983. Volume 2: 300pp. 1984. Maidstone, Kent: The Maidstone Osteopathic Clinic.
A compendium of original and edited articles and photographic descriptions with commentary.

1875   Whiting, Clement A. *Public sanitation and other papers*. 336pp. 1916. Los Angeles, California: The A.T. Still Research Institute.

1876   Williams Publishing Co. (editors). *Osteopathy*. About 150pp. 1910. Kansas City, Missouri: Williams Publishing Co.
A compilation of articles by various authors on the treatment of many different conditions by osteopathy.

1877   Woodhall, Percy H. *Intra-pelvic technic or manipulative surgery of the pelvic organ*. 198pp. 1926. Kansas City, Missouri: Williams Publishing Co.
One of the two definitive works on osteopathic gynaecology (the other is by Clark).

1878   Woodhall, P.H. *A manual of osteopathic gynecology*. 228pp. 1902. Nashville, Tennessee: Jno. Rundle and Sons.
Not as good as Woodhall's gynaecological work.

1879   Woodhall, P.H. *Osteopathy: the science of healing by adjustment*. 110pp. n.d. Orange, New Jersey: The American Osteopathic Association.

Chiropractic

1880   Alberta Chiropractic Association (prepared by). *The chiropractic profession in Alberta.* 80pp. 1976. Alberta: Alberta Chiropractic Association.
A monograph on the status of the chiropractic profession in Canada and the United States and specifically, the province of Alberta.

1881   Altman, Nathaniel. *The chiropractic alternative: a spine owner's guide.* 206pp. 1981. Lakemont, Georgia: Tarnheim Press.

1882   American Chiropractic Association. *American Chiropractic Association policies on public health and related matters.* Des Moines, Iowa: American Chiropractic Association.

1883   American Chiropractic Association. *Basic chiropractic procedural manual.* 260pp. 1973. Des Moines, Iowa: American Chiropractic Association.

1884   American Chiropractic Association. *Benefits of chiropractic inclusion in your health and welfare.* 1979. Des Moines, Iowa: American Chiropractic Association.

1885   American Chiropractic Association. *Lecture notes: 1975.* American Chiropractic Convention. Pages not numbered. 1975. Des Moines, Iowa: American Chiropractic Association.
Technical papers.

1886   American Chiropractic Association and The International Chiropractic Association (editors). *Opportunities in a chiropractic career.* 126pp. 1967. New York: Vocational Guidance Manuals.

Written for the prospective chiropractic student; contains information on education and career opportunities in the chiropractic profession.

1887   Anderson, J.G. *Modern chiropractic: Its science and technique*. 65pp. 1975. Northridge, California: By author.
A textbook for the practitioner and student.

1888   Arnholz, Walter W. *The adjustment of spastic muscle*. 83pp. 1949. Privately published by author.

1889   Arnold, Lee A. *Chiropractic procedural examination*. 219pp. 1979. Privately published by author.
A manual.

1890   Bach, Marcus. *The chiropractic story*. 250pp. 1968. Los Angeles, California: De Vorss.
A readable and popular volume.

1891   Balts, George Alexander. *Chiropractor know thyself*. 237pp. 1936. Los Angeles, California: Privately published by author.

1892   Barge, F.H. *Chiropractic technic*. Volume 1: *Tortipelvis*. 142pp. 1980. Volume 2: *Torticollis*. 138pp. 1979. Volume 3: *Scoliosis*. 328pp. 1981. Davenport, Iowa: Bawden.
Textbooks for the student of chiropractic.

1893   Beatty, Homer G. *Anatomical adjustive technic*. 334pp. 1939. Denver, Colorado: By author.
A textbook and reference book.

1894   Betge, Giorgio. *Physical therapy in chiropractic practice*. 72pp. 1975. Lugano, Switzerland: By author.
Written for the practitioner of chiropractic.

1895   Biron, W.A., B.F. Wells and R.F. Houser. *Chiropractic principles and technic for use by students and practitioners*. 572pp. 1939. Chicago, Illinois: Name of publisher not given.

1896   Brennan, Matthew J. (editor). *The resource guide to chiropractic: a bibliography of chiropractic and related areas*. 155pp. 1981. Washington, D.C.: American Chiropractic Association.
The most comprehensive bibliography of its kind in existence. It is a well-referenced resource base for use by researchers, historians,

librarians, students and interested practitioners. Three thousand listings.

1897   Burich, S.J. *A textbook on chiropractic chemistry*. 430pp. 1919. Davenport, Iowa: By author.

1898   Canadian Memorial College of Chiropractic. *The archives: an anthology of literature relative to the science of chiropractic*. 2 volumes. 572pp. 1974. Toronto, Canada: Canadian Memorial College of Chiropractic.
   An excellent source of reference. A new edition is to be published in 1984.

1899   Canadian Memorial College of Chiropractic. *Segmental neuropathy: the first evidence of developing pathology*. Pages not numbered. n.d. Toronto, Canada: Canadian Memorial College of Chiropractic.

1900   Carver, William. *Carver's chiropractic analysis of chiropractic principles as applied to pathology, relatology, symptomology and diagnosis*. Volume 1. 246pp. n.d. Oklahoma City, Oklahoma: Paul O. Parr. Volume 2 was never written.

1901   Christensen, Kim D. *Illustrated manual of common extremity adjustments*. 71pp. 1980. Privately published by author.

1902   Cleveland, C.S. *Chiropractic principles and practice: outline*. 4 volumes. 1951. Privately published by author.
   An important textbook for students.

1903   Coggis, William N. *Basic technique: a system of body mechanics*. 35pp. 1975. Florissant, Missouri: ELCO.

1904   Commission of Inquiry into Chiropractic in New Zealand. *Chiropractic in New Zealand: the report of the Commission of Inquiry*. 377pp. 1979. Wellington, New Zealand: P.D. Hasselberg, Government Printer.
   Looks at all aspects of chiropractic in New Zealand.

1905   Committee of Inquiry into Chiropractic, Osteopathy, Homoeopathy and Naturopathy. *Report of the Committee of Inquiry into Chiropractic, Osteopathy, Homoeopathy and Naturopathy*. 925pp. 1977. Canberra, Australia: Australian Government Publishing Service.
   Looks at alternative health care in Australia.

1906   Craven, J.H. *A textbook on chiropractic orthopody*. 399pp. 1922. Davenport, Iowa: By author.

1907   Dejarnette, Bertrand. *Chiropractic first aid*. 63pp. 1979. Nebraska City, Nebraska: By author.
A helpful manual that the lay person could use with a little training. Also of use to the practitioner in emergencies.

1908   Dejarnette, B. *Sacro-occipital technique manual*. 256pp. 1982. Nebraska City, Nebraska: Nebraska City Press.

1909   Deloe, Paul. *Preparation of narrative reports for the chiropractic profession*. Pages not numbered. 1980. Garden Grove, California: National Graphics.
An aid to writing professional narrative reports for the practitioner.

1910   Dintenfass, Julius. *Chiropractic: a modern way to health*. 189pp. 1973. New York: Pyramid Publications.
A good overview of the subject for the lay reader.

1911   Dryburgh, Robert. *So you're thinking of going to a chiropractor*. 1984. New Canaan, Connecticut: Keats.
An informative handbook for the prospective patient.

1912   Dye, A. Aug. *The evolution of chiropractic: its discovery and development*. 343pp. 1969. New York: Richmond Hall. This is a photo-reprint of the 1939 edition.

1913   Failor, R.M. *The new era chiropractor*. 88pp. 1979. Palmer Desert, California: By author.

1914   First Research Corporation. *A study and analysis of the treatment of sprain and strain injuries in industrial cases*. 1960. Davenport, Iowa: International Chiropractic Association.

1915   Foundation for Chiropractic Education and Research, The. *Chiropractic health care*. 115pp. 1976. Des Moines, Iowa: The Foundation for Chiropractic Education and Research.

1916   Garsia, Willoughby. *The original 'chiropractic' spinal manipulation*. 228pp. n.d. London: Truth Health.

1917   Gates, Douglas. *Spinal palpation*. 101pp. 1981. Privately published by author.
A textbook and reference work for students.

176

1918   Gertler, Larry. *Illustrated manual of extravertebral technic for students and doctors*. 121pp. 1978. Privately published by author.

1919   Giacomo, F.P. De. *Chiropractic analysis through palpation*. 192pp. 1980. New York: New York Chiropractic College.

1920   Giacomo, F.P. De. *Man's greatest gift to man: chiropractic*. 1970. New York: Parker Publishing Company.

1921   Gillet, H. and M. Liekens. *Belgian chiropractic research notes*. 111pp. 1981. Huntington Beach, California: Motion Palpation Institute.

1922   Gitelman, R., G.G. Murdoch, B.E. Embree and V.G. Dyck (editors). *The archives: an anthology of literature relative to the science of chiropractic*. Volume 1: *Index*. 255pp. Volume 2: *Abstracts*. Pages not numbered. 1984. Toronto, Canada: Canadian Memorial College of Chiropractic.

1923   Gonstead Chiropractic Science and Art. No title. 276pp. n.d. Privately published by the author.
    An important textbook for students. Covers all aspects of chiropractic in twenty chapters.

1924   Grecco, Michael A. *Chiropractic technic illustrated*. 223pp. 1953. New York: Jarl.

1925   Grove, A.B. *Chiropractic technique: a procedure of adjusting*. 131pp. 1979. Madison, Wisconsin: Straus.
    A manual for the practitioner and student.

1926   Haldeman, Scott. *Modern developments in the principles and practice of chiropractic*. 390pp. 1980. New York: Appleton-Century-Crofts.

1927   Harper, W.D. *The principles of chiropractic: anything can cause anything*. 209pp. 1974. San Antonio, Texas: By author.

1928   Hearon, Kevin G. *What you should know about extremity adjusting*. 43pp. 1981. Privately published by author.
    A book for the chiropractor.

1929   Higbe, Denton N. *Spinal analysis: motion palpation.* 75pp. n.d. O'Fallon, Missouri: Professional Books.
Higbe was an early chiropractor.

1930   Higley, Henry G. *The inter-vertebral disk syndrome.* 1965. Des Moines, Iowa: American Chiropractic Association.

1931   Hildebrandt, Roy W. *Chiropractic spinography: a manual of technology and interpration.* 317pp. 1980. Wheaton, Illinois: M.S. Hilmark.

1932   Holmes, Arthur T. *Malpractice as applied to chiropractors.* 253pp. n.d. Privately published by author.

1933   Homewood, A.E. *The chiropractor and the law.* 290pp. 1965. Toronto, Canada: Chiropractor Publishers.

1934   Homola, Samuel A. *Bonesetting, chiropractic and cultism.* 1963. Panama City, Florida: Crique Books.

1935   Homola, S.A. *A chiropractor's treasury of health secrets.* 224pp. 1970. Englewood Cliffs, New Jersey: Prentice-Hall.
Describes self-help programmes for a variety of ailments.

1936   Illi, Fred W. *The vertebral column.* 119pp. 1951. Lombard, Illinois: National College of Chiropractic.
A reference manual.

1937   Inman, O. (editor). *Basic chiropractic procedural manual.* 1973. Des Moines, Iowa: American Chiropractic Association.

1938   International Chiropractic Association (compilers). *Independent studies of industrial back injuries.* 60pp. 1973. Des Moines, Iowa: American Chiropractic Association.

1939   International Chiropractic Association. *International Chiropractic Association manual.* 1979. Davenport, Iowa: By author.

1940   International Chiropractic Association. *Modern developments in the principles and practice of chiropractic.* 1979. New York: Appleton-Century-Crofts.
Consists of a collection of papers given at the Anaheim Conference of 1979. The papers describe current research studies in many areas of chiropractic.

1941 Irvine, Kay (editor). *Index to chiropractic literature.* 147pp. Published annually since 1980. USA: Chiropractic Library Consortium.
Provides a comprehensive subject index to all chiropractic journals published.

1942 Janse, Joseph (edited by Roy W. Hildebrandt). *Principles and practice of chiropractic: an anthology.* 333pp. 1976. Lombard, Illinois: National College of Chiropractic.
A textbook for students.

1943 Janse, J., R.H. Houser and B.F. Wells. *Chiropractic principles and technic for use by students and practitioners.* 660pp. 1978. Lombard, Illinois: National College of Chiropractic.
A standard textbook for students and practitioners. First published in 1947

1944 Jaquet, Pierre. *Clinical chiropractic: a study of cases.* 212pp. 1978. Grounauer, Geneva: By author.

1945 Jaquet, P. *An introduction to clinical chiropractic.* 209pp. 1976. Privately published by author.

1946 Joseph, Max. *Live again with chiropractic.* 188pp. 1980. Mitcham, Surrey: Graphicset.

1947 Kelner, Merrijoy, Oswald Hall and Ian Coulter. *Chiropractors: do they help?* 303pp. 1980. Toronto, Canada: Fitzhenry and Whiteside.

1948 Klein, Lawrence and Sharon Meyer. *Chiropractic: an international bibliography.* 90pp. 1976. Des Moines, Iowa: The Foundation for Chiropractic Education and Reearch.
A review of the world's literature dealing with chiropractic and manipulative therapy. A useful book for researchers in the field.

1949 Larry, James M. and Robert S. Deachman. *A chiropractor's aid to history taking, physical and spinal examinations.* 64pp. 1966. Privately published by authors.
Intended as a guide for newly qualified chiropractors and students.

1950 Leach, Robert A. *The chiropractic theories: a synopsis of scientific research.* 262pp. 1980. Mississippi: Mid-South Scientific Publishers.

An account of the pros and cons of each chiropractic theory with substantial references. A valuable contribution.

1951　Leach, R.A. *The science of chiropractic: its principles and adjustment.* 1980. Davenport, Iowa: The Palmer School of Chiropractic.

1952　Levine, Mortimer. *Structural approach to chiropractic.* 1964. New York: Comet.

1953　Loban, Joy M. *Technic and practice of chiropractic.* 438pp. 1922. Pittsburgh, Pennsylvania: Loban Publishing Co.

1954　McKeon, L.C. Floyd. *A healing crisis.* 175pp. 1933. Weston-super-Mare, Avon: Michell Health Products.

1955　Mawhiney, R.B. *Scoliosis manual.* 68pp. 1982. Waukesha, Wisconsin: Roberts Publications.
A manual for the practitioner.

1956　Maynard, Joseph E. *Healing hands: the official biography of the Palmer family, discoverers and developers of chiropractic.* 407pp. 1977. Mobile, Alabama: Jonorm Publishers.

1957　Medsker, Dennis L. and Paula A. Medsker. *Chiropractic and pediatrics.* 116pp. 1979. Davenport, Iowa: Chiropractic Educational Services.

1958　Morreim, G.M. (edited by Philip W. Hughes). *Pure chiropractic technic.* Pages not numbered. 1975. Privately published by author.
For the practitioner.

1959　Müller, R.O. *Autonomics in chiropractic: the control of the autonomic imbalance.* 189pp. 1975. Toronto, Canada: The Chiropractic Publishing Company.
A practical guide for the chiropractic clinician. A synthesis of information from over a decade of study and application.

1960　Palmer, B.J. *Audiometric changes under specific chiropractic.* 1938. Davenport, Iowa: The Palmer School of Chiropractic.

1961　Palmer, B.J. *Chiropractic clinical controlled research.* 744pp. 1951. Davenport, Iowa: The Palmer School of Chiropractic.

1962　Palmer, B.J. *The chiropractor's adjuster: a compilation of the writings of D.D. Palmer.* 913pp. 1921. Davenport, Iowa: The Palmer School of Chiropractic.

1963   Palmer, B.J. *Electrocardiograph changes under specific chiropractic.* 1938. Davenport, Iowa: The Palmer School of Chiropractic.

1964   Palmer, B.J. *Evolution or revolution.* 126pp. 1957. Davenport, Iowa: The Palmer School of Chiropractic.

1965   Palmer, B.J. *Hermatological changes under specific chiropractic.* 1938. Davenport, Iowa: The Palmer School of Chiropractic.

1966   Palmer, B.J. *The known man, or: an explanation of 'the phenomena of life'.* 341pp. 1936. Davenport, Iowa: The Palmer School of Chiropractic.

1967   Palmer, B.J. *The law of cause and cure of disease, or: the law of production and reduction of vertebral subluxation.* 73pp. 1942. Privately published by author.

1968   Palmer, B.J. *The philosophy of chiropractic.* 428pp. 1920. Davenport, Iowa: The Palmer School of Chiropractic.

1969   Palmer, B.J. *Precise, posture constant spinograph comparative graphs.* 1938. Davenport, Iowa: The Palmer School of Chiropractic.

1970   Palmer, B.J. *The subluxation specific: the adjustment specific.* 870pp. 1934. Davenport, Iowa: The Palmer School of Chiropractic.

1971   Palmer, B.J. *Textbook on the Palmer technique of chiropractic.* 531pp. 1920. Davenport, Iowa: The Palmer School of Chiropractic.

1972   Palmer College of Chiropractic, The. *Manual of chiropractic sciences.* Pages not numbered. 1966. Davenport, Iowa: The Palmer School of Chiropractic.

1973   Palmer College of Chiropractic, The. *Specific spinal correction.* 78pp. 1968. Davenport, Iowa: The Palmer School of Chiropractic.

1974   Palmer, David D. *The chiropractor's adjustor: textbook of the science, art and philosophy of chiropractic.* 1007pp. 1910. Portland, Oregon: Portland Printing House Company.
   Written by the founder of chiropractic, this book examines the practice of chiropractic and its history.

1975   Palmer, D.D. *Three generations: a brief history of chiropractic.* 59pp. 1967. Davenport, Iowa: The Palmer School of Chiropractic.

1976   Reinert, Otto C. *Chiropractic procedure and practice*. 332pp. 1976. Florissant, Missouri: Marian Press.

1977   Rozeiu, Alfred. *A guide to chiropractic research*. 92pp. n.d. Toronto, Canada: Canadian Memorial Chiropractic College.

1978   Schafer, R.C. *Chiropractic health care*. 120pp. 1979. Des Moines, Iowa: The Foundation for Chiropractic Education and Research.

1979   Schafer, R.C. (editor). *Basic chiropractic procedural manual emphasizing geriatric considerations*. Pages not numbered. 1978. Des Moines, Iowa: American Chiropractic Association.

1980   Schafer, R.C. (editor). *Chiropractic: state of the art*. 28pp. 1978. Des Moines, Iowa: American Chiropractic Association.
   Written for the chiropractor.

1981   Schafer, R.C. (editor). *Chiropractic physical spinal diagnosis*. Pages not numbered. 1980. Oklahoma City, Oklahoma: Associated Chiropractic Academic Press.

1982   Schultz, August L. *Athletic and industrial injuries of the foot and ankle*. 191pp. 1958. Mitchell, South Dakota: By author.

1983   Schultz, A.L. *Athletic and industrial injuries of the knee*. 131pp. 1973. Privately published by author.

1984   Schultz, A.L. *The knee, femur and pelvis*. 246pp. 1979. Mitchell, South Dakota: By author.

1985   Schultz, A.L. *The shoulder, arm and hand syndrome*. 279. 1969. Privately published by author.

1986   Schwan, Douglas. *Adjusting the extremities*. 262pp. 1982. Privately published by author.
   A reference manual.

1987   Schwartz, Herman S. (editor). *Mental health and chiropractic: a multidisciplinary approach*. 300pp. 1973. New York: Sessions Publishers.
   A collection of articles that inquire into the legitimacy of the chiropractic role in the field of mental health.

1988   Scofield, Arthur G. *Chiropractic: the science of specific spinal adjustment*. 197pp. 1982. Wellingborough, Northamptonshire: Thorsons.
   Recommended.

1989   Sherman College of Straight Chiropractic. *Specific adjusting contacts*. 87pp. 1978. U.S.A.: Sherman College of Straight Chiropractic.

1990   Simmons, Dean F. *The chiropracto-legal story*. 175pp. 1973. Tacome, Washington: Graphic.

1991   Smith, Ralph Lee. *At your own risk: the case against chiropractic*. 1969 New York: Trident Press.

1992   Spector, Bertram, Leo Eilbert, Fujie Fukuda and Karin Nystrom. *Manual of procedures for moiré contourography*. Part 1: *Administration procedures*. 29pp. Part 2: *A scoring manual*. 29pp. 1979. New York: New York Chiropractic College.
   For the practitioner.

1993   States, Alfred Z. *Atlas of chiropractic technic: spinal and pelvic technics*. 120pp. 1968. Lombard, Illinois: National College of Chiropractic.

1994   Stephenson, R.W. *Chiropractic textbook*. 1948. Davenport, Iowa: The Palmer School of Chiropractic.
   Of historical interest.

1995   Stewart, D.D. *Fundamentals of motion palpation*. 32pp. 1977. Privately published by author.
   A manual.

1996   Stierwalt, D.D. *Adjusting the child*. 67pp. 1976. Davenport, Iowa: By author.

1997   Stierwalt, D.D. *Extremity adjusting*. 38pp. 1976. Davenport, Iowa: By author.

1998   Toftness, I.N. *A look at chiropractic spinal correction: philosophy of chiropractic correlation*. 99pp. 1977. Cumberland, Wisconsin: By author.

1999   Turner, Chittenden. *The rise of chiropractic*. 1931. Los Angeles, California: Powell Publishing Co.

2000   Weiant, C.W. and S. Goldschmidt. *Medicine and chiropractic*. 129pp. 1959. New York: By author.

Chinese Medicine

2001   American Herbal Pharmacology Delegation. *Herbal pharmacology in the People's Republic of China. A trip report (June 1974) of the American Herbal Pharmacology Delegation.* 274pp. 1975. Washington, D.C.: National Academy of Sciences Printing and Publishing Office.

2002   Beau, G. *Chinese medicine.* 190pp. 1972. New York: Avon Books.
A general review of Chinese medicine including a comprehensive section describing the principles of acupuncture.

2003   Chang, Stephen T. *Burn disease out of your body.* 144pp. 1984. Wellingborough, Northamptonshire: Thorsons.

2004   Chen, Ronald. *The history and methods of physical diagnosis in classical Chinese medicine.* 1969. New York: Vantage Press.

2005   Cheung, C.S. and Yat-Ki Lai. *Principles of dialectical differential diagnosis and treatment of traditional Chinese medicine: current interpretation.* 82pp. 1982. San Francisco, California: Traditional Chinese Medicine.
An important and original contribution to the medical diagnosis and treatment system offered by traditional Chinese herbal medicine.

2006   Cheung, C.S. (compiler). *Rationale and correct organisation of prescription of traditional Chinese medicine.* 56pp. 1980. San Francisco, California: Traditional Chinese Medical Publisher.

2007   Cheung, C.S., U. Aik Kaw and Howard Harrison (compilers). *Treatment of toxic side effects resulting from radiation and chemotherapy by traditional Chinese medicine.* 40pp. 1980. San Francisco, California: Traditional Chinese Medical Publisher.

2008 Dimond, E. Gray. *More than herbs and acupuncture.* 223pp. 1975. New York: W.W. Norton.
A very readable account of the author's experiences in China.

2009 Flaws, Bob. *Hit medicine: Chinese medicine in injury management.* 102pp. 1983. Boulder, Colorado: Blue Poppy Press.
Hit medicine applied to Western sports injuries. Readable and interesting.

2010 Fulder, Stephen. *The Tao of medicine: ginseng, oriental remedies and the pharmacology of harmony.* 328pp. 1980. New York: Destiny Books.

2011 Hiller, S.M. and J.A. Jewell. *Health care and traditional medicine in China, 1800–1982.* 472pp. 1983. London: Routledge and Kegan Paul.
A good introduction to an interesting period in the history, development and present practice of Chinese medicine.

2012 Hsu, Hong-Yen (edited by Judith Haueter). *Chinese herbal science: its characteristics, diagnosis and treatment.* 80pp. 1982. Los Angeles, California: Oriental Healing Arts Institute.

2013 Hsu, H. *Chinese herbs and formulas.* 82pp. 1978. Taiwan: Modern Drug Publishing Co.

2014 Hsu, H. (edited by Judith Haueter). *For women only: Chinese herbal formulas.* 203pp. 1982. Los Angeles, California: Oriental Healing Arts Institute.
Many herbal remedies for complaints specific to women.

2015 Hsu, H. *How to treat yourself with Chinese herbs.* 315pp. 1980. Los Angeles, California: Oriental Healing Arts Institute.
Includes disorders and prescriptions.

2016 Hsu, H. *The way to good health with Chinese herbs.* 230pp. 1982. Los Angeles, California: Oriental Healing Arts Institute.
Symptoms and their treatment.

2017 Hsu, H., Yuh-Pan Cheng and Mina Hong. *The chemical constituents of oriental herbs.* 1551pp. 1982. Los Angeles, California: Oriental Healing Arts Institute.
A textbook.

2018   Hsu, H. and Douglas H. Easer. *A practical introduction to major Chinese herbal formulas.* 109pp. 1980. Los Angeles, California: Oriental Healing Arts Institute.

2019   Hsu, H. and Chau-Shin Hsu. *Commonly used Chinese herb formulas with illustrations.* 683pp. 1980. Los Angeles, California: Oriental Healing Arts Institute.
Describes 367 formulas.

2020   Hsu, H. and William Peacher. *Chen's History of Chinese medical science.* 148pp. 1977. Taiwan: Modern Drug Publishers.

2021   Hsu, H. and W.G. Peacher. *Chinese herb medicine and therapy.* 223pp. 1976. Los Angeles, California: Oriental Healing Arts Institute.
An authoritative and detailed discussion.

2022   Huard, Pierre and Ming Wong. *Chinese medicine.* 56pp. 1968. London: Weidenfeld and Nicolson.
A historical text.

2023   Hume, Edward Hicks. *The Chinese way in medicine.* 167pp. 1940. Baltimore, Maryland: Johns Hopkins University Press.

2024   Jain, K.K. *Amazing story of health care in new China.* 184pp. 1973. Emmaus, Pennsylvania: Rodale.
Presents an overview of all aspects of medical care in China today.

2025   Keyes, John D. *Chinese herbs: the botany, chemistry and pharmacodynamics.* 388pp. 1981. Rutland, Vermont: Charles E. Tuttle. First published in 1976.
An illustrated encyclopaedia of more than 250 herbs.

2026   Kushi, Michio. *How to see your health: book of Oriental diagnosis.* 160pp. 1983. Tokyo: Japan Publications.
Covers the principles of diagnosis.

2027   Kushi, M. (edited by William Tara and David Lasock). *Your face never lies: what your face reveals about you and your health. An introduction to Oriental diagnosis.* 82pp. 1983. Wayne, New Jersey: Avery Publishing Group.

2028   Lavier, J. *Chinese micro-massage: acupuncture without needles*. 93pp. 1980. Wellingborough, Northamptonshire: Thorsons.
Bridges the gap between classical massage and acupuncture.

2029   Leslie, Charles (editor). *Asian medical systems: a comparative study*. 419pp. 1976. London: University of California Press.
Focus is on the evolution of ancient medical systems in India, China, the Middle East and Europe and the present structure of knowledge and theory in those areas.

2030   Li, C.P. *Chinese herbal medicine*. 128pp. 1974. Washington, D.C.: U.S. Government Printing Office.
A detailed and technical report.

2031   Lu, H.C. *The Chinese classics of tongue diagnosis in color*. 187pp. 1980. Vancouver, British Columbia: The Academy of Oriental Heritage.
A definitive text on Chinese tongue diagnosis.

2032   Manaka, Y. and I.A. Urquhart. *Quick and easy Chinese massage: pain control and first aid*. 31pp. n.d. San Francisco, California: Japan Publications Trading Co.

2033   Matsumoto, Kiiko and Stephen Birch. *Five elements and ten stems: Nan Ching theory, diagnostics and practice*. 247pp. n.d. Higganum, Connecticut: Paradigm Publications.
A scholarly introduction based on the classical Chinese texts.

2034   Ming, O. (executive editor). *Chinese–English glossary of common terms in traditional Chinese medicine*. 331pp. 1982. Hong Kong: Joint Publishing Co.
Eight thousand entries covering every aspect of Chinese medicine.

2035   Nakamura, Takashi. *Oriental breathing therapy*. 160pp. 1980. Tokyo: Japan Publications.

2036   National Academy of Sciences. *Herbal pharmacology in the People's Republic of China*. 269pp. 1975. Washington, D.C.: National Academy of Sciences Printing and Publishing Office.
A highly technical volume.

2037   Needham, Joseph. *Science and civilisation in China*. 5 volumes. 1464pp. 1980. Cambridge: Cambridge University Press.
An authoritative primary source for all those interested in the history of Chinese science.

2038   Palos, Stephan. *The Chinese art of healing*. 251pp. 1982. New York: Bantam Books.
A well written, comprehensive discussion. Covers acupuncture, massage, folk cures, herbal medicine.

2039   Porkert, Manfred. *The essentials of Chinese diagnostics*. 302pp. 1983. Zürich, Switzerland: Acta Medicinae Sinensis.
An erudite treatise on the theory and practice of Chinese medicine.

2040   Porkert, M. *The theoretical foundations of Chinese medicine: systems of correspondance*. 384pp. 1982. London: MIT Press. First published in 1974.
An impressive study of the medicinal, philosophical and philological aspects of traditional Chinese medicine.

2041   Read, Bernard E. *Chinese medicinal plants from the Pen Ts' Ao Kang Mu. 1596, of a botanical, chemical and pharmacological reference list*. 889pp. 1982. Taipei, Taiwan: Southern Materials Center, Inc.

2042   Revolutionary Health Committee of Hunan Province (prepared by). *A barefoot doctor's manual*. 372pp. 1978. London: Routledge and Kegan Paul.
Used to 'improve the medical and health care facilities in the rural villages' by the use of lay people.

2043   Serizawa, Katsusuke. *Massage: the Oriental method*. 78pp. 1972. San Francisco, California: Japan Publications Trading Co.
The definitive work on Oriental massage.

2044   Shih-Chen, Li (translated and researched by F. Porter Smith and G.A. Stuart). *Chinese medicinal herbs*. 505pp. 1976. San Francisco, California: Georgetown Press. Originally published in 1578.
Includes 1,892 species of herbs and 8,160 prescriptions, and was the product of twenty-six years of research.

2045   Toguchi, Masaru. *Oriental herbal wisdom: a modern guide to the history, traditions, treatment and present practice of the world's most ancient form of healing*. 141pp. 1977. New York: Pyramid Publications.
A good presentation for the general reader.

2046   Veith, Ilza (translator). *The Yellow Emperor's classic of internal medicine*. 260pp. 1972. London: University of California Press. First published in 1949.

Gives an excellent picture of early Chinese medicine, and is an essential work for anyone studying oriental medicine. Includes an introductory study.

2047   Wade, Carlson. *Health secrets from the Orient.* 239pp. 1973. Bergenfield, New Jersey: New American Library.
A survey.

2048   Wallnofer, Heinrich and Anna von Rottauscher (translated by Marion Palmedo). *Chinese folk medicine.* 176pp. 1972. New York: Mentor.
A fascinating account of Chinese medicine and folklore.

2049   Wong, K. Chi Min and Wu Lienteh. *History of Chinese herbal medicine.* 1936. Shanghai, China: National Quarantine Service.

2050   Wong, Pau (editor and translator). *Modern Chinese massotherapy.* 211pp. 1979. Hong Kong: Medicine and Health Publishing Co.
Covers techniques of massage, the acupuncture points used and clinical treatments covered.

2051   Wu, Shui Wan. *The Chinese pulse diagnosis.* 1972. Los Angeles, California: By author.
A pamphlet reviewing various techniques used in conducting traditional Chinese pulse diagnosis.

Acupuncture

2052 Aggrawal, A.L. and G.N. Sharma. *Clinical practice of acupuncture.* 456pp. 1980. Raipur, India: Acupuncture Association of India.
A comprehensive guide.

2053 Akabane, Kobei, Lee Ying-Arng and Wong Chun-Ying. *Method of intracutaneous needles.* 114pp. 1975. Hong Kong: Unicorn Press.
A technical book.

2054 American Anesthesia Study Group. *Acupuncture anesthesia in the People's Republic of China. A trip report.* 73pp. 1976. Washington, D.C.: National Academy of Sciences Printing and Publishing Office.
This report was submitted to the Committee on Scholarly Communication with the People's Republic of China Printing and Publishing Office.

2055 Austin, Mary. *Acupuncture therapy: the philosophy, principles and methods of Chinese acupuncture.* 192pp. 1982. Wellingborough, Northamptonshire: Turnstone Books. First published in 1974.
A comprehensive textbook that is intended as a teaching guide.

2056 Beijing, Shanghai and Nanjing Colleges of Traditional Medicine. *The essentials of Chinese acupuncture.* 445pp. 1980. Beijing, China: Foreign Languages Press. Originally published in 1975 as *An outline of Chinese acupuncture.*
The best 'points' book available, and an essential purchase for any practitioner.

2057 Bischko, Johannes (translated by Diana Reese-Soltész). *An*

introduction to acupuncture. 124pp. 1978. Heidelberg, W. Germany: Karl F. Haug.
One of the most popular introductory books for the student of acupuncture.

2058   Bourdiol, René J. *Auriculosomatology.* 264pp. 1983. Moulins-lès-Metz, France: Maisonneuve.
A textbook.

2059   Bourdiol, R.J. *Elements of auriculotherapy.* 365pp. 1982. Moulins-lès-Metz, France: Maisonneuve.
Written as a definitive text, to clear the misunderstandings in this new field.

2060   Bresler, D.E. *Free yourself from pain.* 1979. New York: Simon and Schuster.

2061   Bresler, D.E., R.J. Kroenig and M.P. Volen. *Acupuncture: can it help?* 1977. Pacific Palisades, California: Centre for Integral Medicine.
A booklet providing answers to questions most commonly asked about acupuncture therapy.

2062   Chaitow, Leon. *The acupuncture treatment of pain.* 160pp. 1979. Wellingborough, Northamptonshire: Thorsons.
Geared to practitioners.

2063   Chan, Pedro. *Acupuncture, electro-acupuncture, anaesthesia.* 44pp. 1972. Alhambra, California: Borden Publishing Company.
An introductory work.

2064   Chan, P. *Wonders of Chinese acupuncture.* 133pp. 1973. Alhambra, California: Borden Publishing Company.
A concise monograph.

2065   Chang, I-Lok and N. Macon (translated by Elliot Silverstein), *Acupuncture and moxibustion.* 1979. New York: Schocken Books.
A handbook for the barefoot doctors of China.

2066   Chang, Stephen Thomas. *The Chinese book of acupuncture.* 264pp. 1976. Berkeley, California: Celestial Arts.
Aimed at the practitioner and the lay person. Covers philosophy and practice.

2067   Chen, James Y.P. *Acupuncture anesthesia in the People's Republic of*

China. 1973. Washington, D.C.: United States Department of Health, Education and Welfare.

2068   Cheng-wei, Lee (editor and translator). *The manual of China's current acupuncture therapy*. 247pp. 1981. Hong Kong: Medicine and Health Publishing Co.
Suitable for acupuncturists, physicians and those who are interested in the subject. First published in 1975.

2069   Cheong, W.C. and C.P. Yang. *Synopsis of Chinese acupuncture*. 131pp. 1976. Hong Kong: The Light Publishing Co.
A well presented summary for the practitioner and a useful introduction for the layman.

2070   China Cultural Corporation. *Acupuncture charts*. 4 charts. 1975. Hong Kong: Toppan Printing.

2071   Chu, Luke S.W., Samuel D.J. Yeh and Denise D. Wood. *Acupuncture manual: a Western approach*. 272pp. 1979. New York: Marcel Dekker.
Includes history, modern developments and research.

2072   College of Chinese Medicine, Peking (edited by Torben Clausen). *Practical acupuncture: an illustrated intoduction*. 160pp. 1973. Copenhagen: Fadl.
A good overall handbook meant for the Chinese health worker in his study of acupuncture.

2073   Colleges of Traditional Chinese Medicine of Beijing, Shanghai and Nanjing and the Acupuncture Institute of the Academy of Traditional Chinese Medicine (compilers). *Essentials of Chinese acupuncture*. 456pp. n.d. Beijing: Foreign Languages Press.

2074   Connelly, Dianne M. *Traditional acupuncture: the law of five elements*. 200pp. 1979. Columbia, Maryland: Center for Traditional Acupuncture.

2075   Cooperative Group of Shandong Medical College and Shandong College of Traditional Chinese Medicine, The. *Anatomical atlas of acupuncture points*. 265pp. 1982. Jinan, China: Shangdong Science and Technology Press.
Descriptions as well as illustrations of the courses of the channels and location of the points.

ALTERNATIVE MEDICINE

2076　Duke, Marc. *Acupuncture*. 283pp. 1973. London: Constable.
A detailed introductory work for the lay person and student.

2077　Ewart, Charles. *The healing needles*. 118pp. 1972. London: Elm
Tree Books.

2078　Graystone, Peter and James Lymell. *Acupuncture and pain
therapy: comprehensive bibliography*. 1975. Vancouver: Biomedical
Engineering Services.

2079　Gwei-Djen, Lu and Joseph Needham. *Celestial lancets: history
and rationale of acupuncture and moxa*. 427pp. 1980. Cambridge:
Cambridge University Press.
A detailed historical account of the techniques of acupuncture and
moxa. The only book of its kind in a Western language.

2080　Hashimoto, Masae (edited and annotated by Philip M.
Chancellor). *Japanese acupuncture*. 80pp. 1968. London: Thorsons.

2081　Heroldová, Dana (compiler and translator). *Acupuncture and
moxibustion*. 2 parts with supplement: Charts and illustrations. 1968.
Prague, Czechoslovakia: Oriental Institute in Academia, Publishing
House of the Czechoslovak Academy of Sciences.
Translations of modern Chinese texts.

2082　Ho, S.T. and L.K. Lu (compiler and translator). *The principles
and practical use of acupuncture anaesthesia*. 350pp. 1981. Hong Kong:
Medicine and Health Publishing Co. First published in 1974.
A technical, but readable, book.

2083　Huang, Helena. *Ear acupuncture*. 149pp. 1972. Emmaus,
Pennsylvania: Rodale.

2084　Hwang, Paul T.K., S.L. Joshua and Pedro C.P. Chen.
Acupuncture made easy. 1975. Alhambra, California: Chan's Books.

2085　Jayasuriya, A. *Acupuncture therapeutics*. 193pp. 1979. Fernardo,
Sri Lanka: Lake House Publishing.
A valuable book for all students and practitioners of acupuncture.

2086　Jayasuriya, A. *Clinical acupuncture*. 355pp. 1979. Fernardo, Sri
Lanka: Lake House Publishing.
An elementary book written mainly as a guide to the barefoot
doctors of the world, but still a useful reference work.

2087   Jayasuriya, A. and Felix Fernando. *Principle and practice of scientific acupuncture.* 479pp. 1978. Fernardo, Sri Lanka: Lake House Publishing.
Contains a clear statement of theory and a step-by-step approach to the application of acupuncture.

2088   Jenerick, H.P. *Proceedings—NIH Acupuncture Research Conference.* 1973. Bethesda, Maryland: National Institutes of Health.
Contains summary research reports.

2089   Jiasan, Yang (editor). (translated by Meng Xiankun and Li Xuewu). *The way to locate acu-points.* 74pp. 1982. Beijing, China: Foreign Languages Press.
Takes anatomical landmarks as criteria for locating points.

2090   Kaptchuk, Ted J. *The web that has no weaver.* 402pp. 1983. London: Rider and Co.
An excellent introduction to the principles of Chinese medicine.

2091   Kenyon, Julian N. *Modern techniques of acupuncture. A practical scientific guide to electro-acupuncture.* Volume 1: 240pp. Volume 2: 108pp. 1984. Volume 3: Towards a new approach to medicine. 250pp. To be published April 1985. Wellingborough, Northamptonshire: Thorsons.
A scientific account of European developments in electro-acupuncture and its relationship to classical Chinese acupuncture.

2092   Kho, L.K. (compiler and translator). *How to apply face, nose, hand and foot acupuncture.* 57pp. 1981. Hong Kong: Medicine and Health Publishing Co.
Gives the points, needling methods and prescriptions.

2093   Kinoshita, Haruto. *Illustration of acupoints.* 36pp. 1970. Tokyo: Ido-No-Nippon-Sha.

2094   Kurashima, S. *Circulatory disease, renal bladder diseases, skin diseases.* 125pp. 1976. Kanagawo, Japan: Ido-No-Nippon-Sha.

2095   Kurashima, S., Lee Ying-Arng and Wong Chun-Ying. *Circulatory diseases (hypertension, hypotension and tachycardia, etc.)* 94pp. 1977. Hong Kong: Unicorn Press (No. 6 in the *Modern Acupuncture and Moxibustion* series.)

2096   Kwok-Chi, Yau. *The treatment of bronchial asthma by the Chinese medical practice of 'Bu Shen' (tonification of the kidney) and acupuncture therapy.* 10pp. 1977. Hong Kong: Chinese Medicine Publications.

2097   Kwong, Lo Chi. *Nose, hand and foot acupuncture.* 46pp. 1981. Hong Kong: The Commercial Press. First published in 1976. Introductory text on the points, indications for their use and needling methods by the Chairman of the International Acupuncture Society in Hong Kong.

2098   Lavier, J. (translated and edited by Philip Chancellor). *Points of Chinese acupuncture.* 116pp. 1979. Holsworthy, Devon: Health Science Press. A helpful revision guide for students and reference guide for practitioners.

2099   Lawson-Wood, D. and J. Lawson-Wood. *Acupuncture handbook.* 151pp. 1964. Rustington, Sussex: Health Science Press. An early textbook for students and practitioners which presents a Westernized form of the science.

2100   Lawson-Wood, D. and J. Lawson-Wood. *Five elements of acupuncture and Chinese massage.* 107pp. 1966. Rustington, Sussex: Health Science Press. A concise introductory work on traditional five-element acupuncture. Recommended.

2101   Lawson-Wood, D. and J. Lawson-Wood. *The incredible healing needles.* 63pp. 1974. New York: Samuel Weisner. A good introductory book for the lay reader.

2102   Lawson-Wood, D. and J. Lawson-Wood. *Multilingual atlas of acupuncture. 17 colour plates of anatomical drawings of the major acupuncture points as they are located on the body.* 1967. Rustington, Sussex: Health Science Press.

2103   Lee, J.F. and C.S. Cheung. *Current acupuncture therapy.* 408pp. 1978. Hong Kong: Medical Book Publications. A comprehensive text.

2104   Leger, Jean-Paul. *The little red book of acupuncture.* 64pp. 1982. Wellingborough: Thorsons. First published in 1978. A simply written guide to the basic principles of acupuncture.

2105   Leong, Lucille. *Acupuncture: a layman's view.* 139pp. 1974. Bergenfield, New Jersey: New American Library.
An overview of acupuncture.

2106   Leonhardt, H. *Fundamentals of electro-acupuncture according to Voll: an introduction.* 248pp. 1980. Uelzen, W. Germany: M.L. Verlag.
Aims to show how to diagnose safely and quickly.

2107   Lewith, George T. *Acupuncture: its place in Western medical science. An introduction to, and an explanation of this Eastern system of medicine.* 127pp. 1982. Wellingborough, Northamptonshire: Thorsons.

2108   Lewith, G.T. and N.R. Lewith. *Modern Chinese acupuncture: a review of acupuncture techniques as practised in China today.* 144pp. 1983. Wellingborough, Northamptonshire: Thorsons.

2109   Low, R. *The secondary vessels of acupuncture: a detailed description of the meridians of acupuncture, beyond the 12 principal ones.* 192pp. 1983. Wellingborough, Northamptonshire: Thorsons.

2110   Lowe, William C. *Introduction to acupuncture anaesthesia.* 107pp. 1973. London: Henry Kimpton.

2111   Lowenkopf, Anne N. *Osteopuncture: relief from strong and chronic pain.* 196pp. 1976. Santa Barbara, California: Medical Arts.
Describes what osteopuncture is, and what it can do.

2112   Lu, Henry C. *Chinese acupuncture for pain relief.* 291pp. 1974. Vancouver, British Columbia: The Academy of Oriental Heritage.
Looks at Chinese theories of pain, and the clinical differentiation of pain diagnosis and relief.

2113   Lu, H.C. *A complete textbook of auricular acupuncture.* 319pp. 1975. Vancouver, British Columbia: The Academy of Oriental Heritage.
A translation of materials published in the 1970s from the Zoological Research Institute of The Chinese Academy of Sciences and People's Public Health Press, Beijing.

2114   Lu, H.C. *Scalp acupuncture: therapy and anaesthesia.* 110pp. 1975. Vancouver, British Columbia: The Academy of Oriental Heritage.
Describes a new branch of acupuncture, scalp acupuncture, including twenty-three diseases which it is being used to treat in China.

2115 Lu, H.C. *The true story of Chinese acupuncture.* Volume 1: 331pp. Volume 2: 223pp. 1979. Vancouver, British Columbia: The Academy of Oriental Heritage.
Covers the full range of Chinese acupuncture for the educated layman and doctor.

2116 Lu, H.C. (translator). *The Yellow Emperor's Classic of Internal Medicine and the difficult classic.* 5 volumes. 1978. Vancouver, British Columbia: The Academy of Oriental Heritage.
Gives Chinese and English texts, though no commentary.

2117 Macdonald, Alexander. *Acupuncture: from ancient art to modern medicine.* 184pp. 1984. London: Unwin.
An invaluable guide for patient and practitioner, which provides authoritative and comprehensive answers to the most common questions.

2118 McGarey, William. *Acupuncture and body energies.* 146pp. 1974. Phoenix, Arizona: Gabriel Press.
A readable and balanced view of how acupuncture fits into Western medical thought.

2118A Man, Pang L. *Handbook of acupuncture analgesia.* 1973. Woodbury, New Jersey: Field Place Press.

2119 Manaka, Yoshio and Ian Urquhart. *The layman's guide to acupuncture.* 143pp. 1972. New York: Weatherhill.
A thorough introduction to acupuncture.

2120 Mann, Felix Bernard. *Acupuncture: cure of many diseases.* 128pp. 1980. London: William Heinemann Medical Books.
Briefly surveys many aspects of the theory and practice of acupuncture.

2121 Mann, F.B. *Acupuncture: the ancient Chinese art of healing.* 212pp. 1980. London: William Heinemann Medical Books. First published in 1962.
Recommended.

2122 Mann, F.B. *Atlas of acupuncture.* 1981. London: William Heinemann Medical Books. First published in 1966.
Three charts relating points and meridians to surface anatomy.

2123   Mann, F.B. *The meridians of acupuncture.* 174pp. 1981. London: William Heinemann Medical Books. First published in 1964.
A detailed account.

2124   Mann, F.B. *Scientific aspects of acupuncture.* 106pp. 1983. London: William Heinemann Medical Books.
Written for doctors as 'an attempt to describe acupuncture in terms of science'.

2125   Mann, F.B. *The treatment of disease by acupuncture.* 224pp. 1980. London: William Heinemann Medical Books. First published in 1963.
An instructive book. Describes two different departures for treatment.

2126   Marcus, Paul. *Acupuncture: a patient's guide.* 112pp. 1984. Wellingborough, Northamptonshire: Thorsons.
An introductory guide for the layman.

2127   Margutti, Victor M. *Acupuncture biodynamic energies and homoeopathy: a therapeutic étude.* 251pp. 1982. New Delhi: B. Jain.
A mixture of acupuncture, homoeopathy, Bach remedies, tissue salts and Indian classical medicine, showing how they interrelate.

2128   Matsumoto, Teruo. *Acupuncture for physicians.* 203pp. 1974. Springfield, Illinois: Charles C. Thomas.
A very technical survey of the clinical practice of acupuncture.

2129   Matsumoto, T. and Bruce A. Levy. *Acupuncture for patients.* 107pp. 1975. Springfield, Illinois: Charles C. Thomas.

2130   Medicine and Health Publishing Company. *China's new needling treatment.* 92pp. 1979. Hong Kong: Medicine and Health Publishing Co.
A textbook.

2131   Medicine and Health Publishing Company. *An explanatory book of the newest illustrations of acupuncture points.* 113pp. 1981. Hong Kong: Medicine and Health Publishing Co.
A detailed study.

2132   Medicine and Health Publishing Company. *The latest chart of auricular points.* 1983. Hong Kong: Medicine and Health Publishing Company.

2133   Medicine and Health Publishing Company (edited and translated by Lee Cheung-Wei). *The manual of China's current acupuncture therapy.* 247pp. 1981. Hong Kong: Medicine and Health Publishing Company. First published in 1975.
Covers eight kinds of acupuncture techniques, the 151 commonly used acupuncture points and fifty-seven common diseases and treatments. It is 'suitable for acupuncturists, physicians and those interested in the subject'.

2134   Medicine and Health Publishing Company. *Practical ear-needling therapy.* 162pp. 1982. Hong Kong: Medicine and Health Publishing Co.
An introductory textbook to auriculotherapy.

2135   Medicine and Health Publishing Company. *The treatment of 100 common diseases by new acupuncture.* 89pp. 1980. Hong Kong: Medicine and Health Publishing Co.
In table form. Very clear and easy to follow. Interesting for the general reader but also a useful symptomatic reference book for the practitioner.

2136   Meeran, Munsif. *Acupuncture, science and art.* 64pp. 1984. London: Mehar Printers.
Written as a simple introduction for patients, doctors and medical students. Covers new techniques.

2137   Mori, Hidetaro. *Diseases of locomotor apparatus.* 52pp. 1973. Yokosuka, Japan: Ido-No-Nippon-Sha. (Volume 3 of the *Modern acupuncture and moxibuxtion* series).

2138   Mori, H. (translated by Judy Craig). *Introductory acupuncture: Japanese acupuncture technique and treatment.* 175pp. 1977. Tokosuka, Japan: Ido-No-Nippon-Sha.
A student's guide to Goushin, the use of fine needles, techniques of insertion, withdrawal, etc.

2139   Moss, Louis. *Acupuncture and you.* 196pp. 1972. London: Paul Elek Books. First published in 1964.
A description of acupuncture and its application to the treatment of rheumatism, by a practising MD.

2140   Nakatani, Yoshio. *A guide for application of Ryodoraku autonomous nerve regulating therapy.* 25pp. 1972. Alhambra, California: Chan's Books.
A technical study.

2141   Nakatani, Y. and Kumio Yamashita. *Ryodoraku acupuncture. A guide for the application of Ryodoraku therapy: electrical acupuncture, a new autonomic nerve regulating therapy.* 207pp. 1977. Tokyo, Japan: Ryodoraku Research Institute.
The definitive work on the subject. Describes the differences between this new therapy and classical acupuncture.

2142   Nogier, P.F.M. (translated by Helena Huang). *Ear acupunture.* 150pp. 1974. Emmaus, Pennsylvania: Rodale.

2143   Nogier, P.F.M. *From auriculotherapy to auriculomedicine.* 231pp. 1983. Moulins-lès-Metz, France: Maisonneuve.
Meant as an introduction to ear therapy (discovered only twenty-five years ago).

2144   Nogier, P.F.M. (translated by Julian Kenyon). *Handbook to auriculotherapy.* 163pp. 1981. Moulins-lès-Metz, France: Maisonneuve.
An introduction for practitioners.

2145   Nogier, P.F.M. *Treatise of auriculotherapy.* 321pp. 1972. Moulins-lès-Metz, France: Maisonneuve.
A classic of the French school.

2146   Omura, Yoshiaki. *Acupuncture medicine: its historical and clinical background.* 287pp. 1982. Tokyo, Japan: Japan Publications.
A textbook.

2147   Paine, David L.S. *Acupuncture: traditional diagnosis and treatment.* 99pp. 1984. London: East Asia Co.
A short introduction for the doctor and other health practitioners to Chinese acupuncture from the traditional point of view.

2148   Peking Foreign Language Press. *Acupuncture anaesthesia.* 26pp. 1972. Beijing, China: Foreign Languages Press.

2149   People's Medical Publishing House. *Advances in acupuncture and acupuncture anaesthesia: abstracts of papers presented on the National Symposium of Acupuncture, Moxibustion and Acupuncture Anaesthesia, Beijing, June 1–5 1979.* 541pp. 1980. Beijing, China: The People's Medical Publishing House.
A technical work.

2150   Player, Graham. *Disease and diagnosis for the acupuncturist: an advanced guide to traditional diagnostic techniques.* 142pp. 1984. Wellingborough, Northamptonshire: Thorsons.
An advanced guide for practitioners of acupuncture, based on the traditional Chinese theories of medicine.

2151   Research Institute of Chinese Traditional Medicine of Peking with Medical Workers. *'Plum blossom' needle therapy.* 70pp. 1982. Hong Kong: Medicine and Health Publishing Company.
Covers the history and therapeutic uses of this technique.

2152   Robinson, Nicola and Monty Berman. *Acupuncture and general practice: a radical view.* 74pp. 1984. London: East Asia Co.
An account of a research project: the effects of introducing acupuncture into general practice using a non-medical acupuncturist.

2153   Roberts, Michael J. *Acupuncture therapy: its mode of action.* 17pp. 1981. Leicester: Eresus Publications.

2154   Rose-Neil, Sidney. *Acupuncture and the life energies.* 160pp. 1981. New York: ASI Publishers.
A personal description and explanation of the history, philosophy and theory of Ch'i involved in acupuncture.

2155   Rose-Neil, S. *An acupuncturist visits China.* 192pp. 1979. London: The British Acupuncture Association.
Based on the author's diary during his visit to China as a guest of the Academy of Traditional Medicine, Beijing.

2156   School of Traditional Medicine, Beijing (translated by the Acupuncture Research Institute). *Acupuncture made easy. A clinical reader.* 95pp. 1975. Alhambra, California: Chan's Books.
A classic textbook.

2157   Serizawa, K. *Tsudo-vital points for Oriental therapy.* 256pp. 1976. Tokyo, Japan: Japan Publications.
A broad and detailed account.

2158   Shanghai Academy of Traditional Chinese Medicine. (compilers). *Anatomical charts of acupuncture points and fourteen meridians.* Set of 6 charts. Shanghai, China: Shanghai Academy of Traditional Chinese Medicine.

2159   Shanghai College of Traditional Medicine (translated and edited by John O'Connor and Dan Bensky). *Acupuncture: a comprehensive text.* 740pp. 1981. Chicago, Illinois: Eastland Press.
An authoritative reference and source book on acupuncture both ancient and modern.

2160   Silverstein, M.E., I. Iok Chang and Nathaniel Macon (translators). *Acupuncture and moxibustion.* 118pp. 1975. New York: Schocken Books.
Handbook used by the barefoot doctors in the People's Republic of China.

2161   Stiefvater, Eric H.W. *What is acupuncture? How does it work?* 47pp. 1971. Holsworthy, Devon: Health Science Press.
Brief introduction to acupuncture.

2162   Tam, Billy K.S. and Miriam S.L. Tam. *Acupuncture: an international bibliography.* 137pp. 1973. Metuchen, New Jersey: The Scarecrow Press.

2163   Tan, T. Leong, Margaret You-Ching Tan and Ilza Veith. *Acupuncture therapy: current Chinese practice.* 172pp. 1976. London: Routledge and Kegan Paul.
A technical book for practitioners and doctors.

2164   Toguchi, Masaru. *The complete guide to acupuncture.* 1974. Wellingborough, Northamptonshire: Thorsons.
A comprehensive handbook geared to the general reader who wishes to become a practitioner.

2165   Turner, Roger Newman and Royston H. Low. *The principles and practice of moxibustion: a guide to the therapeutic application of heat to acupuncture points.* 95pp. 1981. Wellingborough, Northamptonshire: Thorsons.
A comprehensive guide for the practitioner.

2166   Voison, Henry (translated by Herman Kamenetz). *Essentials of acupuncture.* 1976. 159pp. Quebec: Edisem. First published in France in 1950.

2167   Voll, Reinhold. *Inter-relations of odontons and tonsils to organs, fields of disturbance, and tissue systems.* 179pp. 1978. Uelzen, West Germany: M.L. Verlag.
A theoretical work dealing with the approved remote effects originating from odontogenous foci based on classical acupuncture.

2168   Voll, R. (translated and revised by Hartwig Schuldt). *Topographic positions of the measurement points in electro-acupuncture.* 6 volumes. 1968. Uelzen, W. Germany: M.L. Verlag.

2169   Wae, Shui. *A research into acupuncture and its clinical practice.* 231pp. 1977. Hong Kong: The Commercial Press.
The result of forty years of research and clinical experience by the author.

2170   Warren, Frank Z. *Handbook of medical acupuncture.* 273pp. 1976. New York: Van Nostrand Reinhold.

2171   Warren, F.Z. and Theodore Berland. *The acupuncture diet.* 136pp. 1976. New York: St. Martin's Press.
The effectiveness of ear needling or ear-stapling acupuncture for weight loss.

2172   Warren, F.Z. and Walter I. Fischman. *Sexual acupuncture.* 248pp. 1978. New York: Dutton.
A clear discussion of recent findings of acupuncture for sex problems.

2173   Warren, F.Z. and Helena L. Huang. *Ear acupuncture.* 1974. Emmaus, Pennsylvania: Rodale.

2174   Wei-Kang, Fu. *Chinese acupuncture and moxibustion.* 1975. Beijing, China: Foreign Languages Press.

2175   Wei-Ping, Wu. *Chinese acupuncture.* 181pp. 1974. Wellingborough, Northamptonshire: Thorsons.
Essentially a textbook for practitioners who wish to follow the classical Chinese tradition.

2176   Wensel, Louise Oftedal. *Acupuncture in medical practice.* 335pp. 1980. Reston, Virginia: Reston Publishing Co.
Looks at the status, role and use of acupuncture in present-day North America.

2177   Werner, Fritz (translated by Hartwig Schuldt). *Electro-acupuncture primer.* 164pp. 1979. Ulzen, W. Germany: Medizinisch-Literarische Verlagsgesellschaft.
An introductory manual.

2178   Wexu, Mario. *The ear, gateway to balancing the body: a modern guide to ear acupuncture.* 203pp. 1975. New York: ASI Publishers.
General introductory textbook.

2179   Woollerton, Henry and Colleen J. McLean. *Acupuncture energy in health and disease: a practical guide for advanced students.* 126pp. 1983. Wellingborough, Northamptonshire: Thorsons.

2180   Worsley, J.R. *Is acupuncture for you?* 82pp. 1973. Leamington Spa: The College of Traditional Chinese Acupuncture, U.K.
A good introductory work written in a question-and-answer format.

2181   Worsley, J.R. *The acupuncturist's therapeutic pocket book.* 200pp. 1975. Columbia, Maryland: The Center For Traditional Acupuncture.

2182   Worsley, J.R. *Everyone's guide to acupuncture.* 93pp. 1974. London: Cassell and Co.
Describes what happens at a visit to an acupuncturist, how to train to be an acupuncturist and what acupuncture is good for.

2183   Worsley, J.R. *Law of five elements.* Leamington Spa, Warwickshire: The College of Traditional Chinese Acupuncture, U.K.
A set of four anatomical charts describing the meridians of energy which govern the practice of acupuncture.

2184   Worsley, J.R. *The meridians of Ch'i energy: points reference guide.* 8pp. 1979. Tisbury, Wiltshire: Element Books.

2185   Worsley, J.R. *Talking about acupuncture in New York.* 112pp. 1982. Tisbury, Wiltshire: Element Books.
Transcript of a seminar given in New York to a lay audience.

2186   Worsley, J.R. *Traditional Chinese acupuncture.* Volume 1: *Meridians and points.* 327pp. 1982. Tisbury, Wiltshire: Element Books.
A reference work for students and practitioners.

2187   Yanagiya, S. (translated by F.G.T. Carrodus). *Family secret one-needle acupuncture.* 63pp. n.d. London: The British Acupuncture Association. First published in Japanese in 1948.
Deals with the basic therapy called by the Chinese 'Nei Ching'.

2188   Yau, P.S. (editor and translator). *Scalp-needling therapy.* 72pp. 1980. Hong Kong: Medicine and Health Publishing Co.

A new technique of the 1970s, used for example in the treatment of paralysis and Ménière's disease.

2189   Yue-sun, Sung. *Chi Kung and acupuncture*. 20pp. n.d. Hong Kong: Tsimshatsui.
Meditation exercises related to acupuncture for clearing the mind.

Index

References are to item numbers, not pages.

Colitis 942, 1170
Colon 1043, 1131, 1233, 1365, 1373
Comfrey 622
Congenital defects 95, 111
Constipation 140, 591, 734, 983,
1026, 1256, 1260, 1438
Constitutional medicine 131
Consumption 100, 112, 223, 397
Cosmotherapy 1430
Cystitis 1139, 1212, 1331

Dandelions 702
Deficiency diseases 412
Depression 105, 1663, 1664
Diabetes 199, 324, 819, 900, 1638,
1649
Diarrhoea and dysentery 40, 127,
128, 484
Digestion and indigestion 54, 71,
142, 248, 543, 712, 878, 883, 1149,
1267
Domestic medicine 133, 165, 167,
225, 261, 280, 284, 336, 337, 375,
450, 531, 532, 582, 610, 611, 618,
619, 1004, 1044
Drainage 329
Duodenum 69, 711, 1417

Ears and hearing 436, 1414, 1729,
1748, 2083, 2142, 2173, 2178
Electro-homoeopathy 220
Emergencies and accidents 76, 123,
216, 464, 497, 1764
Emotional health 443, 920, 1354,
1468, 1575
Emphysema 820, 1329, 1330
Enzymes 883, 1089, 1471
Epilepsy 437
Evening primrose oil 1582, 1637
Eyes and sight 93, 334, 354, 626,
844, 845, 846, 850, 851, 954, 974,
1007, 1062, 1201, 1202, 1203,
1220, 1301, 1324, 1348, 1359,
1380, 1408, 1409, 1439, 1748

Fasting 889, 899, 909, 910, 911, 957,
958, 979, 1001, 1034, 1073, 1125,
1207, 1211, 1215, 1253, 1289,
1361, 1396, 1397, 1405

Fever 16, 23, 102, 205, 485
Fistula 109
Fluoridation 904, 1039
Foxglove 785

Gall bladder 1035, 1459
Gall stones 104, 711
Garlic 518, 731
Genetotrophic concept 1508
Ginseng 573, 583, 585, 603, 606,
609, 614, 625, 2010
Glands 53, 135, 144, 654, 1378
Glandular medicines 7
Goitre 984
Gold 105
Gout 106
Grape cure 890, 1391
Gunpowder 139
Gynaecology 163, 472, 1721, 1824,
1877, 1878

Hahnemann, Samuel 81, 99, 157,
177, 178, 237, 247, 264, 270, 273,
355, 459, 465, 481
Hair 3, 542, 1285, 1415, 1421, 1444,
1545, 1594, 1642
Hay fever 1024, 1266, 1454, 1500
Headaches and migraine 592, 932,
1002, 1195, 1216, 1273, 1363
Heart 105, 118, 136, 243, 364, 593,
654, 703, 714, 886, 936, 1137,
1164, 1270, 1437, 1440, 1443,
1455, 1540, 1576, 1636, 1638,
1641, 1668, 1675, 1679
Herbal medicine 246, 387, 498–791
Herbal teas 536, 537, 538, 570, 600
Hernia 943, 1171
Homoeopathy 1–497, 951, 1722,
1905, 2127
Honey 849, 889, 913, 1055, 1276,
1364
Hypoglycaemia 794, 801, 810, 838,
891, 901, 1022, 1183, 1491
Hypothyroidism 839

Indigestion, see Digestion and indigestion
Influenza 74, 130, 590, 821, 1050,
1643

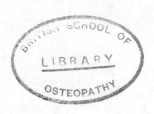